Clinical Approaches to Tachyarrhythmias

edited by

A. John Camm, MD

Volume 15

Clinical Approaches to Tachyarrhythmias (CATA)
Series Editor: A. John Camm, MD

Volume 1. **Mechanisms of Arrhythmias**
by *Michiel J. Janse, MD*

Volume 2. **Electrocardiographic Diagnosis of Tachycardias**
by *Clifford J. Garratt, MA, MD, Michael J. Griffith, MA, MD*

Volume 3. **Risk Assessment of VentricularTachyarrhythmias**
by *Mark H. Anderson, MD*

Volume 4. **Atrial Fibrillation for the Clinician**
by *Francis D. Murgatroyd, MA, A. John Camm, MD*

Volume 5. **ICD Therapy**
by *Karl-Heinz Kuck, MD, Riccardo Cappato, MD, Jürgen Siebels, MD*

Volume 6. **The Wolff-Parkinson-White Syndrome**
by *Carlos A. Morillo, MD, George J. Klein, MD, Raymond Yee, MD, Gerard M. Guiraudon, MD*

Volume 7. **The Long QT Syndrome**
by *Peter J. Schwartz, MD*

Volume 8. **Ventricular Tachyarrhythmias in the Normal Heart**
by *John P. Bourke, MD, J. Colin Doig, MB*

Volume 9. **Clinical Aspects of Implantable Cardioverter-Defibrillator Therapy**
by *Martin Fromer, MD*

Volume 10. **The Brugada Syndrome**
by *Charles Antzelevitch, PhD, Pedro Brugada, MD, PhD, Josep Brugada, MD, PhD, Ramon Brugada, MD, Koonlawee Nademanee, MD, Jeffrey Towbin, MD, PhD*

Volume 11. **Atrial Tachycardia**
by *Michael D. Lesh, MD, Franz X. Roithinger, MD*

Volume 12. **QT Dispersion**
by *Marek Malik, PhD, MD, DSc*

Volume 13. **Catheter Ablation of Ventricular Tachycardia in Patients with Structural Heart Disease**
by *Martin Borggrefe, MD, Thomas Wichter, MD, Günter Breithardt, MD*

Volume 14. **Atrial Flutter: From Mechanism to Treatment**
by *Albert L. Waldo, MD*

CLINICAL APPROACHES TO TACHYARRHYTHMIAS
edited by
A. John Camm, MD
St. George's Hospital Medical School
London, United Kingdom

Volume 15

Arrhythmias in Heart Failure
by

William G. Stevenson, MD

Laurence M. Epstein, MD

William H. Maisel, MD

Michael O. Sweeney, MD

Lynne W. Stevenson, MD

The Cardiovascular Division
Department of Medicine
Brigham and Women's Hospital
Harvard Medical School
Boston, Massachusetts

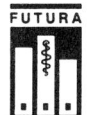

Futura Publishing Company, Inc.
Armonk, NY

SOUTH UNIVERSITY
709 MALL BLVD.
SAVANNAH, GA 31406

Library of Congress Cataloging-in-Publications

Arrhythmias in heart failure / William G. Stevenson ... [et al.].
  p. ; cm. — (Clinical approaches to tachyarrhythmias ; v. 15)
Includes bibliographical references and index.
ISBN 0-87993-707-6 (alk. paper)
  1. Arrhythmia. 2. Heart failure. I. Stevenson, William G., MD. II. Series.
[DNLM: 1. Arrhythmia—complications. 2. Heart Failure, Congestive—
etiology. WG 330 C6403 1993 v. 15]
RC685.A65 A7785 2002
616.1'28—dc21

2002017679

Copyright ©2002
Futura Publishing Company, Inc.

Published by
Futura Publishing Company
135 Bedford Road
Armonk, NY 10504
www.futuraco.com

LC#: 2002017679
ISBN#: 0-87993-707-6

Every effort has been made to ensure that the information in this book is as up to date and accurate as possible at the time of publication. However, due to the constant developments in medicine, the author, the editors, and the publisher cannot accept any legal or other responsibility for any errors or omissions that may occur.

All rights reserved.
No part of this book may be translated or reproduced in any form without written permission of the publisher.

Printed in the United States of America on acid-free paper.

Foreword

Heart failure is an increasingly common condition, the end result of many different mechanisms and pathologies. Arrhythmias are commonly encountered in the context of heart failure and are due not only to the pathophysiological state of heart failure, but also to the underlying structural heart disease. Two arrhythmias predominate: atrial fibrillation and ventricular tachycardia/fibrillation.

Significant strides have been in the treatment of ventricular arrhythmias, both when patients have already presented with a life-threatening arrhythmia (secondary prevention) and prior to the first such event in patients at high risk of suffering them (primary prevention) by the prescription of an implantable cardioverter defibrillator (ICD). Adjunctive or complementary drug therapy is currently being explored and both amiodarone and sotalol appear to be useful therapies. Frequently, recurrent forms of ventricular tachycardia may also be effectively treated by catheter-based ablation techniques provided that an ICD is also used as a safety net.

Atrial fibrillation has proven more difficult to treat. Anticoagulation is usually needed, provided that serious hemorrhagic complications are not anticipated. The control of the ventricular rate is essential, either by AV nodal blockade with digitalis or beta-blockers, or by suppressing the atrial fibrillation with antiarrhythmic drugs. Specific trials of antiarrhythmic treatment in heart failure with amiodarone and dofetilide suggest benefit in terms of reducing the likelihood of atrial fibrillation and fewer subsequent hospitalizations (dofetilide), but no convincing reduction of mortality has been demonstrated. Rate control does seem to improve depressed left ventricular function and may lead to greater benefit.

In this volume of the *Clinical Approaches to Tachyarrhythmias,* William Stevenson and his colleagues from Boston summarize for the practicing physician and cardiologist the current management of arrhythmias in patients with heart failure. It has not been usual for the etiology of arrhythmias to greatly influence the treatment of the condition but there are very many particular features about the arrhythmias that occur in the setting of heart failure that the etiology is relevant to the mechanism and management of the condition. "Upstream" therapy has been pioneered in this clinical arena—treatment of the underlying heart disease and the hemodynamic abnormalities have resulted in a substantial reduction in the arrhythmia burden.

The aim of this series of monographs devoted to cardiac arrhythmology, made possible with assistance of an educational grant from Medtronic, Inc., is to update the physician and cardiologist and all of those responsible for caring for patients with cardiac arrhythmias about the spectacular developments in diagnostic and interventional cardiac electrophysiology.

A. John Camm, MD
Professor of Clinical Cardiology
St. George's Hospital
London, United Kingdom

Preface

It is perhaps surprising that the prevalence of heart failure is increasing despite better care and outcomes for patients with coronary artery disease and hypertension. In part, this reflects the aging population and longer survival of patients with heart disease. The frequency of cardiac arrhythmias, both life-threatening ventricular arrhythmias and atrial fibrillation, parallels the severity of heart failure. Therapies that benefit heart failure by blunting neurohormonal responses are likely to reduce arrhythmias, but the extension of survival achieved may be shifting the clinical presentations to a later age. As heart failure management has progressed so has our understanding of arrhythmias in heart failure and of the impact of arrhythmia therapies. For many clinical scenarios, a rational management strategy has emerged. As important as establishing therapies that should be implemented is the recognition of therapies that, although seemingly rational at one point in time, are now recognized as having greater potential for harm, such as Class I sodium channel blocking antiarrhythmic drugs.

Clinicians will continue to be confronted with vexing arrhythmia management problems in this patient population. Who should receive an implanted defibrillator? Should we be screening for arrhythmia risk markers? When are attempts to maintain sinus rhythm better than simply controlling the ventricular response during atrial fibrillation? Good approaches to many clinical situations are established from clinical trials. For other problems, reasonable management options can generally be formulated based on our present knowledge base, although randomized trials are not yet available. In either case, when confronting an individual patient, a variety of issues particular to that patient's situation need to be considered and management individualized.

This monograph attempts to provide the clinician with current fundamentals of arrhythmias in heart failure as they relate to a variety of clinical scenarios. Although a simple strategy for decision making cannot always be derived, we hope that clinicians will find the information useful for assessing and managing arrhythmias and arrhythmia risk in their patients with heart failure.

William G. Stevenson, MD

Contents

Foreword v
Preface vii

1. Arrhythmias and Heart Failure: Relation to
   Heart Failure Syndromes and Sudden Death 1
2. Use of Antiarrhythmic Drugs in Heart Failure 12
3. Implantable Defibrillators in Heart Failure 18
4. The Cardiac Arrest Survivor 32
5. Sustained Ventricular Tachycardia 37
6. Primary Prevention of Arrhythmic Sudden Death:
   Nonsustained Ventricular Tachycardia and
   Other Potential Markers of Risk 45
7. Syncope 56
8. Bradyarrhythmias and Pacing 61
9. Atrial Fibrillation and Flutter 70

References 76
Index 103

1

Arrhythmias and Heart Failure:

Relation to Heart Failure Syndromes and Sudden Death

In the United States alone there are more than 4 million patients diagnosed with heart failure. Cardiac arrhythmias are a common and important feature of heart failure that contribute to symptoms, periodic decompensations, and mortality in the form of sudden death. Arrhythmia recognition and management is an important aspect of caring for patients with heart failure. The population of patients with heart failure is diverse, with differences that impact on the incidence of arrhythmias and on diagnostic and therapeutic strategies. Patients with depressed systolic function and ventricular dilation have "chronic dilated heart failure." These patients can be broadly considered as falling into two groups based on the etiology of heart disease (Figure 1–1). Patients with dilated heart failure due to coronary artery disease, commonly referred to as "ischemic cardiomyopathy," typically have had a prior myocardial infarction, with a large area of infarct scar and a remodeled, dilated left ventricle. The large infarct scar is often associated with inducible ventricular tachycardia (VT) at electrophysiologic study (EPS) (see below and Chapter 6). Patients with chronic dilated heart failure due to idiopathic, familial, and post-viral cardiomyopathies, or aortic or mitral regurgitation are commonly referred to as having "nonischemic dilated cardiomyopathies." Patients with nonischemic cardiomyopathy typically lack large areas of ventricular scar; inducible VT at EPS is uncommon. Chronic dilated heart failure from any cause is associated with an increased risk of sudden death. Atrial fibrillation and flutter are also common.

Chronic heart failure symptoms also occur in an increasing number of patients who have preserved systolic function, sometimes referred to as heart failure with diastolic dysfunction. Hy-

2 CLINICAL APPROACHES TO TACHYARRHYTHMIAS

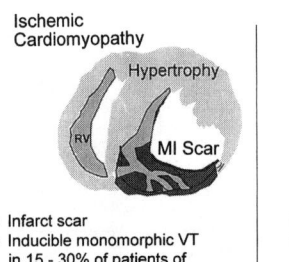
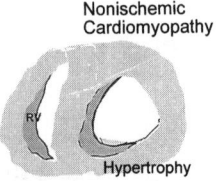

Ischemic Cardiomyopathy	Nonischemic Cardiomyopathy

• Infarct scar
• Inducible monomorphic VT in 15 - 30% of patients of all patients with significantly depressed ventricular function
	• No infarct scar
	• monomorphic VT inducible in fewer than 5 % of patients who do not present with the arrhythmia
	Causes:
	    familial
	    post - viral
	    idiopathic
	    valvular
	    hypertension

• Similar sudden death risk
• Similar efficacy of ICD in sudden death prevention for patients resuscitated from VT/VF

Figure 1–1. Patients with ischemic cardiomyopathy have typically suffered a large myocardial infarction followed by ventricular remodeling. The infarct provides the substrate for potential reentry, causing VT that is typically monomorphic and inducible at EP testing. Myocardial hypertrophy can be present in the surviving remodeled ventricle. Patients with nonischemic cardiomyopathy have ventricular hypertrophy; large confluent areas of scar or infarction are absent in most patients. In unselected patients, monomorphic VT is very infrequent. Those few patients who do present with monomorphic VT usually have inducible VT at EP testing. Despite the differences, both groups are at risk for sudden death.

pertension, advanced age, and diabetes mellitus are common associations. Ventricular arrhythmias are not as well studied in this patient population. The risk of sudden death may be less than that for patients with chronic dilated heart failure. Atrial fibrillation is a major feature of this clinical syndrome and its occurrence is often associated with hemodynamic deterioration.

Links between Ventricular Arrhythmia Mechanisms and Clinical Presentations

Repolarization and Torsades de Pointes

Chronic heart failure is accompanied by ventricular hypertrophy, which is manifest not only as an increase in ventricular mass, but also as cellular hypertrophy, changes in ionic currents, and alterations in the ventricular interstitium (Figure 1–2). Repolarizing potassium currents are reduced, delaying repolarization and prolonging action potential duration. Impaired intracellular calcium handling promotes increased activity of the Na–Ca exchanger, which also contributes to action potential prolongation.[1-7] In the surface electrocardiogram, action potential prolongation is manifest as QT interval prolongation.

These electrophysiologic changes may increase the susceptibility of patients with heart failure to the polymorphic VT torsades de pointes (see Chapter 5, and Figure 5–4), and, in part, the increased risk of drug-induced proarrhythmia in heart failure.[2,8] Potassium and magnesium depletion from chronic diuretic therapy also promotes arrhythmias and torsades de pointes.[9-12] In one series of patients with heart failure, torsades de pointes caused 13% of cardiac arrests.[13,14] Administration of the potassium channel blocking antiarrhythmic drug dofetilide to patients with heart

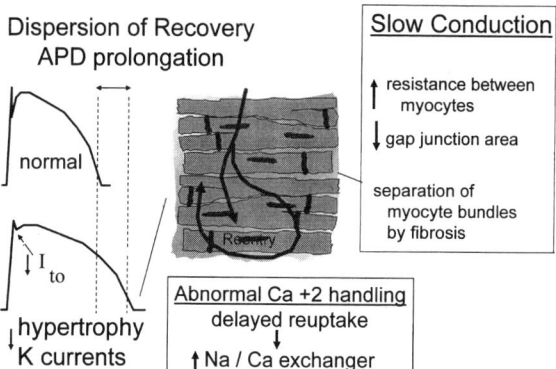

Figure 1–2. The electrophysiologic changes of hypertrophy are summarized.[1-5] Action potential duration is prolonged due to diminished repolarizing potassium currents. In particular, the transient outward current I_{to}, which causes the notch of the action potential, is diminished. Dispersion of recovery is increased. Intercellular coupling is diminished by changes in gap junctions and separation of myocytes and myocyte bundles by interstitial fibrosis. Diminished coupling slows conduction. These changes predispose to reentry. Intracellular calcium handling is abnormal, which, along with action potential prolongation, predisposes to torsades de pointes.

failure was associated with a 5% risk of torsades de pointes or marked QT prolongation even when precautions were taken to exclude susceptible patients.[15] Patients who have had torsades de pointes due to one agent remain at risk for recurrence when exposed to other agents that prolong the QT interval.[8] The potential susceptibility to torsades de pointes warrants several precautions in patients with heart failure. Patients treated with antiarrhythmic drugs that prolong the QT interval (sotalol, dofetilide, quinidine, procainamide, ibutilide, or disopyramide) should have drug therapy initiated in-hospital with electrocardiographic monitoring and careful observation for the occurrence of marked QT prolongation and torsades de pointes (Chapter 2). Amiodarone is an exception, which has a much lower risk of torsades de pointes, and can be safely initiated out of hospital for most patients. Even amiodarone should be avoided, however, in heart failure patients who have had torsades de pointes due to another agent unless they have an implanted defibrillator.[8]

Hypertrophy and Slow Ventricular Conduction

Ventricular hypertrophy in heart failure is associated with slowing of conduction through the myocardium (Figure 1–2). Development of fibrous tissue between myocytes and diminished gap junction surface area decrease cell-to-cell coupling, slowing conduction through the myocardium.[5,16–18] Slow conduction promotes reentrant arrhythmias. Slow conduction is manifest in the surface electrocardiogram as QRS prolongation. Increased QRS duration appears to be a marker for increased mortality in heart failure, although it may reflect more severe ventricular dysfunction and greater myocardial mass, rather than a specific marker for arrhythmia risk.

Ventricular Scars and Infarcts Causing Reentrant Ventricular Tachycardia

Patients with ischemic cardiomyopathy typically have large areas of infarction (Figure 1–1). In some patients, surviving myo-

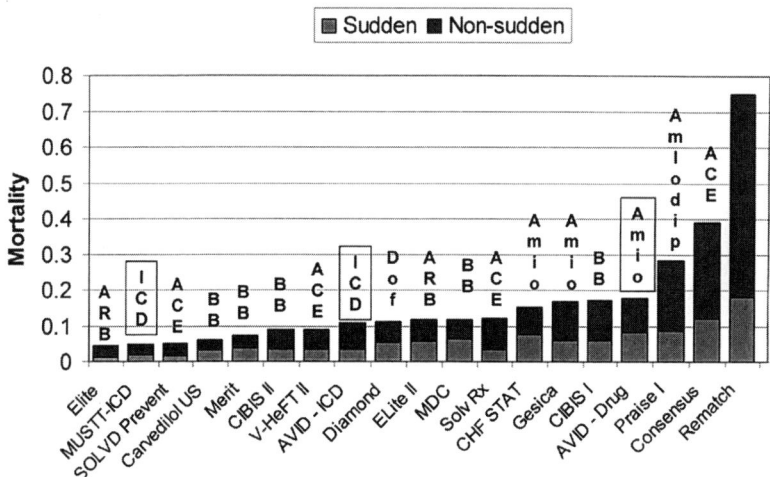

Figure 1–3. Annualized, 1-year total mortality and sudden death (black portion of the bar) from recent heart failure and arrhythmia trials are shown. Mortality is from the treatment group for trials of beta-blockers (BB), angiotensin-converting enzyme inhibitors (ACE) or angiotensin II blockers (ARB), amiodarone (Amio), or ICD. Data from the MUSTT and AVID trials that targeted patients at risk for arrhythmias and not heart failure are indicated by a box around either Amio or ICD. The greatest mortality is from the medical therapy group of the REMATCH trial, which randomized Class IV heart failure patients to medical therapy or a mechanical left ventricular assist device.

cyte bundles are present within the infarction, creating channels for conduction that set up a reentry circuit.[18,19] Interstitial fibrosis involving myocyte bundles in these channels slows conduction, promoting reentry. The VT that results is typically monomorphic, with each QRS complex resembling the preceding and following QRS complex (see Chapter 5). Because the arrhythmia substrate is relatively fixed and stable, tachycardia is usually inducible with programmed stimulation in the electrophysiology laboratory. Electrophysiologic testing can be used to detect the presence of these reentry circuits, thereby identifying patients at risk of spontaneous episodes.

In patients with idiopathic nonischemic cardiomyopathy, large areas of scar or infarction are usually absent (Figure 1–1).

6 CLINICAL APPROACHES TO TACHYARRHYTHMIAS

Programmed stimulation rarely induces sustained monomorphic VT in unselected patients with nonischemic cardiomyopathy.[20,21] Interestingly, of the uncommon patients who develop sustained monomorphic VT, most have evidence of large areas of ventricular scar associated with a reentry circuit.[22] The scar may be a consequence of replacement fibrosis from the myopathic process itself or due to infarcts from embolism of left ventricular or atrial thrombus to a coronary artery. Scars causing VT in the absence of coronary artery disease should prompt consideration of sarcoidosis, Chagas' disease, and arrhythmogenic right ventricular dysplasia.[23-30] Approximately 20% to 40% of patients with monomorphic VT associated with nonischemic cardiomyopathies have reentry through the bundle branches (Chapter 5) causing their VT.[17] This tachycardia is also inducible by programmed stimulation.

Sympathetic Stimulation

Sympathetic stimulation is arrhythmogenic. In heart failure, beat-to-beat heart rate variability and increased circulating catecholamine levels are markers of increased sympathetic tone.[31-35] Sympathetic activation parallels the severity of heart failure and is associated with increased mortality. The risk of sudden death is increased, but not out of proportion to the total increase in mortality.[10,11,31,36,37]

Myocardial Ischemia

Myocardial ischemia also plays a role in promoting arrhythmias and causing sudden death in heart failure.[38] Acute myocardial ischemia can cause polymorphic VT and ventricular fibrillation (VF) (Figure 1-4). Sympathetic activation, hypokalemia, and myocardial hypertrophy increase the risk of developing VF during an episode of myocardial ischemia.[39-41] This potential is well recognized in patients with heart failure associated with coronary artery disease, but the frequency with which it occurs is underappreciated. In a review of 171 autopsies from patients

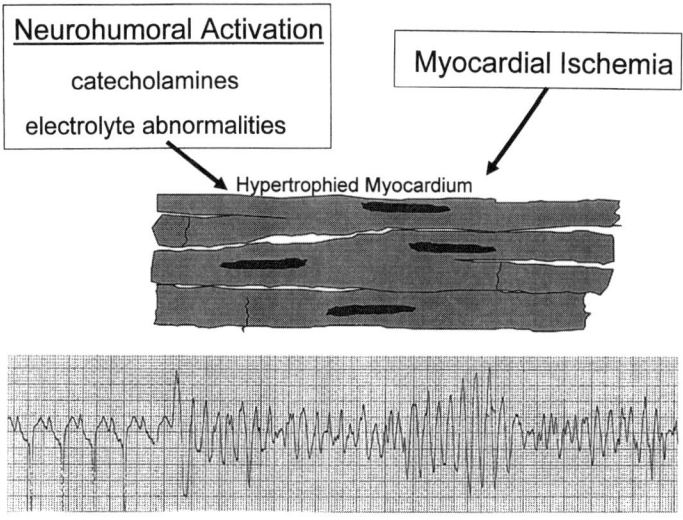

Figure 1–4. The electrocardiogram at the bottom shows initiation of sustained polymorphic VT due to acute myocardial ischemia during a myocardial infarction. Ventricular hypertrophy, hypokalemia, and increased sympathetic tone predispose to development of VF during myocardial ischemia.

who died in one large heart failure trial, 42% of sudden unexpected deaths were associated with acute coronary lesions or evidence of acute myocardial infarction that was usually clinically unsuspected.[38] Unsuspected atherosclerotic coronary artery disease is common in patients who carry a diagnosis of "nonischemic cardiomyopathy."[38] These considerations emphasize the importance of therapies that reduce the risk of ischemia and ischemic arrhythmias in patients with heart failure associated with coronary artery disease. Attention to therapies that reduce the risk of sudden death associated with ischemic heart disease is important in patients with heart failure, especially when coronary artery disease is known or suspected. Such therapies include antiplatelet agents, angiotensin-converting enzyme inhibitors, beta-adrenergic blockers, and lipid-lowering therapies (Table 1–1).[42–45]

Table 1-1

Sudden Death Prevention By Therapies That Do Not Target Arrhythmias

Angiotensin-converting enzyme inhibitors or angiotensin II receptor blockers*
Beta-adrenergic blockers*
Maintenance of potassium homeostasis—prevention of hypokalemia and hyperkalemia
Prevention of hypomagnesemia
Anticoagulation with warfarin for selected patients
    Prior thromboembolic event
    Atrial fibrillation or flutter
    Intracardiac thrombus on echocardiogram
Patients with coronary artery disease
    Assessment and treatment of myocardial ischemia
    Aspirin or clopidogrel for patients with coronary artery disease*
    Lipid-lowering therapy

*Efficacy established by randomized trials. Other therapies are generally recommended and supported by clinical observations.

Electrolyte Abnormalities

Patients with heart failure are predisposed to development of hypokalemia and hypomagnesemia as a consequence of chronic diuretic therapy.[12,39,46,47] Hypokalemia predisposes to torsades de pointes and to VF during myocardial ischemia. The role of hypomagnesemia is less clear, but may also contribute to these arrhythmias and impair repletion of potassium stores.

Impaired renal perfusion, and administration of potassium supplements, angiotensin-converting enzyme inhibitors, angiotensin II receptor blockers, and aldosterone antagonists, can predispose to development of hyperkalemia that can cause sinusoidal VT (see Figure 4–3) or bradyarrhythmias.

Bradyarrhythmias and Electromechanical Dissociation

Although ventricular arrhythmias are likely the major cause of sudden death in heart failure, other mechanisms also occur.[38,48–50] Bradyarrhythmias cause approximately of in-hospital unexpected cardiac arrests.[49,50] Conduction disease associated with heart failure, myocardial ischemia, antiarrhythmic and beta-adrenergic blocking drugs, and hyperkalemia are important causes. Bradyarrhythmias and pulseless electrical rhythm may be more common presentations of cardiac arrest in patients with nonischemic cardiomyopathy as compared to ischemic cardiomyopathy, and in patients hospitalized with advanced heart failure compared to stable out-patients.

Impaired atrioventricular (AV) conduction and interventricular conduction are common in patients with heart failure, generally reflect the severity of the underlying heart disease, and are markers of increased mortality.[51–53] In one series, 28% of 94 patients with nonischemic dilated cardiomyopathy had first- or second-degree AV block on ambulatory electrocardiogram monitoring. Impairment of AV conduction was associated with a greater than 4-fold increase in the risk of sudden death.[53]

When sudden death occurs in a patient who has an implanted defibrillator, electromechanical dissociation and bradycardia pacing are often recorded by the device during the fatal episode.[48,54] Unexpected and unrecognized acute myocardial infarction, pulmonary embolism, stroke, and ruptured aortic aneurysms cause some of these deaths.

Sudden Death in Chronic Dilated Heart Failure

In chronic dilated heart failure, the incidence of sudden death increases with the severity of heart failure (Figure 1–3).[12,34,43,55–61] In patients with minimal to modest symptoms of heart failure (New York Heart Association functional Class I–II), the annual risk of sudden death ranges from 2% to 6% per year. Those with more advanced symptoms (New York Heart Association functional Class III–IV) have a risk of 5% to 12% per year. As the severity of heart failure increases, deaths due to pump failure increase to a greater extent than sudden deaths. Thus, the proportion of deaths that are sudden and unexpected decreases from between 50% and 80% for mild to moderate heart failure to between 5% and 30% for severe heart failure.

It is likely that the majority of sudden deaths are due to VT degenerating to VF (see Figure 3–1). However, as discussed above, the arrhythmia does not occur through the same mechanism in all patients.[38,48,49] In patients with ischemic cardiomyopathy, acute myocardial ischemia and reentry through regions of old infarct scars are most likely. In patients with nonischemic cardiomyopathy, the mechanisms are less well defined, but reentrant VT and polymorphic tachycardias are important causes. The risk of sudden death is approximately similar for a given severity of ventricular dysfunction regardless of whether heart failure is due to ischemic as compared to nonischemic cardiomyopathy.[38,39,62]

Medical therapy for symptomatic dilated heart failure now routinely includes angiotensin-converting enzyme inhibitors and beta-blockers when tolerated. These therapies reduce total mortality. In most cases, it appears that sudden death is reduced in parallel with total mortality. A statistically significant reduction in sudden death is observed in some trials.[43,44,56,63,64] In others, the sample size may not be sufficient to establish statistical significance for that fraction of mortality.

Implications of Multiple Causes of Sudden Death in Heart Failure

Any single intervention will not prevent all causes of sudden death. Implantable cardioverter-defibrillators (ICDs) effectively treat many cardiac arrests due to VT or VF, but if the arrhythmia is due to a large myocardial infarction or hyperkalemia, rather than a primary arrhythmia, or if it occurs in the end-stages of heart failure, the ultimate outcome is likely to be death (see Figure 3–3).

Some interventions that do not specifically target arrhythmias will prevent some sudden deaths (Table 1–1). Preventive therapies for some causes of sudden death are generally accepted, although definitive evidence from randomized trials is not available. Attention to electrolyte balance and avoiding drug toxicities that cause torsades de pointes or bradyarrhythmias is important. Angiotensin-converting enzyme inhibitors and beta-adrenergic blockers reduce sudden death risk; beneficial effects on hypertrophy and reduction of sympathetic activation may play a role.[64,65]

Anticoagulation for patients with a history of prior thromboemboli or other risk factors for emboli, such as atrial fibrillation or ventricular thrombus identified on echocardiogram, is also recommended. Antiplatelet therapy with aspirin or clopidogrel is recommended for patients with coronary artery disease.[66] Lipid-lowering therapy is warranted for patients with coronary artery disease.[67]

2

Use of Antiarrhythmic Drugs in Heart Failure

There are few antiarrhythmic drug options for patients with heart failure. Beta-adrenergic blockers have antiarrhythmic effects and demonstrated efficacy for improving mortality and reducing sudden death.[45,68–70] Beta-blockers can help control the ventricular response to atrial fibrillation and diminish symptoms of palpitations from supraventricular arrhythmias and premature ventricular contractions.[71] Beta-blockers have limited efficacy for many arrhythmias and can aggravate bradyarrhythmias.

Class I Sodium Channel Blocking Antiarrhythmic Drugs

In patients with heart failure, the Class I sodium channel blocking drugs (mexiletine, tocainide, procainamide, quinidine, disopyramide, flecainide, and propafenone) should be avoided. These drugs have negative inotropic effects (with the possible exception of quinidine).[72,73] Blockade of sodium channels diminishes intracellular sodium and thereby diminishes the activity of the sodium–calcium exchanger (the opposite effect of digitalis). Quinidine may lack negative inotropic effects because vasodilation, and QT interval prolongation, which allows additional time for calcium to enter during the plateau phase of the action potential, may offset the negative inotropic effects of the sodium channel blockade. Class I antiarrhythmic drugs also have a potential for proarrhythmia that is likely facilitated by the electrophysiologic changes of heart failure and hypertrophy.[74,75] These adverse effects of Class I antiarrhythmic drugs likely explain the increase in mortality that has been observed when these agents were administered to patients with prior myocardial infarction, to patients with heart failure and atrial fibrillation, and to patients who had been resuscitated from a cardiac arrest.[69,74,76] Thus, the

Class I antiarrhythmic drugs are now largely reserved for control of frequent symptomatic arrhythmias in patients who have an implantable defibrillator and when amiodarone, dofetilide, or sotalol are less attractive options.

Amiodarone

Amiodarone is the major option for antiarrhythmic drug therapy in patients with heart failure, largely because it is relatively safe from a cardiac standpoint.[77–83] Amiodarone blocks cardiac sodium, potassium, and calcium currents and has sympatholytic effects. It has activity against both ventricular and supraventricular arrhythmias. Individual trials have found either a benefit or no effect on mortality.[77,78] A meta-analysis of randomized trials in patients with heart failure concluded that amiodarone reduces mortality by 17% and reduces sudden death by 23%.[80] Whether there is a survival benefit is controversial, but a major adverse impact is unlikely.

Subgroup analysis suggests that amiodarone is more likely to be beneficial for patients with nonischemic cardiomyopathy, and for those who have a relatively elevated resting heart rate ($\geq$90/min) after adjustment of heart failure therapy.[77,78] Chronic therapy with amiodarone slows resting heart rate by approximately 10 beats per minute, which is associated with an improvement of ventricular function, and with an increase in left ventricular ejection fraction of approximately 8 percentage points.[81] Mortality may be improved through this mechanism rather than through any specific antiarrhythmic effect.[81,82]

Ventricular proarrhythmia is unusual with amiodarone. In large heart failure and postmyocardial infarction trials, amiodarone has been initiated in the outpatient setting, without electrocardiographic monitoring, and no increase in mortality was observed.[77,78,80,83] Amiodarone has potent effects on the sinus and AV nodes. Bradyarrhythmias are the major cardiac risk, occurring in approximately 1% to 7% of patients in randomized trials, and in up to a third of patients in some case series.[80–84] Amiodarone should not be administered to patients with marked bradycardia in the absence of a permanent pacemaker.

In patients with compensated heart failure, amiodarone is well tolerated from a hemodynamic standpoint when administered at a loading dose of 600 to 800 mg daily for 1 to 2 weeks.[77–80,83,84] In patients with decompensated heart failure, administration of the loading dose, and in particular large oral doses (e.g., >1200 mg daily) can exacerbate heart failure.[85] The heart rate slows without a compensatory increase in stroke volume.

Noncardiac toxicities are a major problem during therapy with amiodarone. In randomized trials, 41% of patients discontinue therapy by 2 years due to real or perceived side effects. The true incidence of side effects is lower, as indicated by the observation that placebo was discontinued in 27% of patients in these trials.[80] However, it is often difficult to distinguish an amiodarone-induced side effect from symptoms of dyspnea or fatigue related to heart failure. Amiodarone-induced pulmonary toxicity occurs in approximately 1% of patients per year.[86] Chronic therapy at doses exceeding 300 mg per day increases the risk. Patients must be carefully followed for potential toxicities. We obtain liver function tests and a thyroid stimulating hormone (TSH) assay every 6 months during chronic therapy. A chest radiograph should be obtained annually. Annual pulmonary function tests are recommended by some physicians, particularly for those patients taking a daily dose in excess of 300 mg. A decrease in diffusing capacity can indicate development of pulmonary toxicity.[87] When pulmonary toxicity is suspected, a right heart catheterization to assess the possibility of pulmonary vascular congestion and a chest CT scan to assess interstitial fibrosis can be helpful in assessing the contribution of pulmonary toxicity as compared to congestive heart failure.[87,88]

Hyper- or hypothyroidism occurs in up to 18% of patients.[89] Hypothyroidism is easily managed with thyroid replacement therapy and does not generally warrant discontinuation of amiodarone. Hyperthyroidism is a much more difficult problem. Control with antithyroid medications can be difficult. Because the gland is saturated with iodine from the amiodarone, radioactive iodine is not adequately taken up by the gland to allow thyroid ablation. Discontinuation of the drug and medical therapy for hyperthyroidism is often required.

Although amiodarone prolongs action potential duration, often markedly, it rarely causes torsades de pointes. In addition to blocking repolarizing potassium currents, amiodarone also blocks calcium and sodium currents that might play a role in generation of afterdepolarizations causing torsades de pointes. Out-patient antiarrhythmic drug loading with amiodarone is common practice, the safety of which is supported by trials in postmyocardial infarction and heart failure populations.[78,90] However, heart failure patients who have had torsades de pointes in response to any antiarrhythmic agent or perturbation are at high risk for sudden death when treated with amiodarone, suggesting that this group of patients might be particularly susceptible.[8] Of eight patients with advanced heart failure and a history of torsades de pointes before being treated with amiodarone, four died suddenly within 1 year during treatment with amiodarone.[8] Bradycardia prolongs the QT interval and promotes torsades de pointes. Amiodarone-induced bradycardia might be particularly important in causing torsades de pointes in these patients.

Amiodarone increases the energy required for defibrillation and can render an ICD ineffective in some patients (see Chapter 3). It can also impair arrhythmia detection by slowing the rate of VT. These concerns warrant careful testing of ICD function and defibrillation after amiodarone therapy is initiated in patients with ICDs.

Dofetilide

Dofetilide is a Class III antiarrhythmic drug that is approved for therapy of atrial fibrillation.[15] It blocks the repolarizing potassium current I_{Kr}, increasing action potential duration and the QT interval. Its major toxicity is proarrhythmia from torsades de pointes, which occurs in more than 3% of patients.[15] It is excreted largely through the kidney with a plasma half-life of 9.5 hours. When precautions are taken, avoiding administration to patients with prolonged QT intervals or with renal insufficiency, and initiating therapy in-hospital with electrocardiographic monitoring, dofetilide can be administered safely to patients with heart failure. The Danish Investigations of Arrhythmia and Mortality on Dofetilide (DIAMOND) study enrolled 1518 patients who had been hospitalized with Class III or IV heart failure. During a median follow-up of 18 months, there was no difference in mortality between dofetilide-treated and placebo groups.[15] Dofetilide-treated patients were less likely to be rehospitalized for exacerbation of heart failure (30% compared to 38%), possibly due to a reduction in atrial fibrillation during follow-up.

Dofetilide is an antiarrhythmic drug option for selected heart failure patients. It is presently approved only for treatment of atrial fibrillation in the United States. It requires initiation in-hospital with continuous electrocardiographic monitoring for a minimum of 72 hours to detect the development of QT prolongation and torsades de pointes. It should not be administered to patients with significant renal insufficiency (calculated creatinine clearance <20 mL/min).

Sotalol

Sotalol is a Class III drug that, similar to dofetilide, blocks the potassium current I_{Kr}. Unlike dofetilide, sotalol is also a potent nonselective beta-adrenergic blocker. Sotalol has not been specifically evaluated in heart failure patients. In survivors of myocardial infarction who have depressed ventricular function, chronic therapy with the d-isomer of sotalol, which lacks the beta-blocking effect, increases mortality.[91] Sotalol causes torsades de pointes with a similar incidence to that of dofetilide and can aggravate bradyarrhythmias and heart failure through its beta-blocking effects. Therapy should be initiated in-hospital during continuous electrocardiographic monitoring. It also has a renal route of excretion and should be avoided in patients with renal insufficiency. Antiarrhythmic efficacy for atrial fibrillation is less than that of amiodarone.[92]

Summary

In general, antiarrhythmic drug therapy should be avoided. Amiodarone is a reasonable option when symptomatic ventricular arrhythmias or atrial fibrillation require therapy. Dofetilide can be considered for attempted maintenance of sinus rhythm in patients with atrial fibrillation who do not have additional risk factors for torsades de pointes. Other drugs are sometimes useful for diminishing the frequency of arrhythmias in patients who have an ICD.

3
Implantable Defibrillators in Heart Failure

Indications

Implantable cardioverter-defibrillators (ICDs) provide the best available protection from death due to VT or VF (Figure 3–1). The superiority of ICDs to therapy with amiodarone has been convincingly demonstrated for patients who have been resuscitated from a cardiac arrest (Table 3–1, and Chapter 4).[76,93–96] In the Antiarrhythmics Versus Implantable Defibrillator (AVID) trial, total mortality at 3 years was reduced from 36% to 25%, an 11% absolute reduction in mortality and a 31% relative reduction in mortality compared to antiarrhythmic drug therapy (amiodarone in over 95% of patients). Two smaller trials also show similar trends.[76,94,95]

ICDs offer several advantages over antiarrhythmic drug therapy. Provided that the device is functioning properly, compliance is assured and not dependent on patient cooperation. Antiarrhythmic drug toxicities are avoided, unless a drug is required to reduce frequent arrhythmia episodes. ICDs also provide backup bradycardia pacing for treatment of bradyarrhythmias.

In addition to patients who have been resuscitated from a cardiac arrest or sustained VT, ICDs should also be considered for several other groups of patients who have a recognized risk of sudden death from arrhythmias (Table 3–2). ICDs improve survival in patients with coronary artery disease who have depressed left ventricular function (left ventricular ejection fraction ≤ 0.4) with nonsustained VT and inducible VT at EPS (see below). ICDs are also warranted for patients with heart failure and unexplained syncope (Chapter 7), particularly for those with nonischemic cardiomyopathy, and for patients with a familial cardiomyopathy or arrhythmia syndrome associated with sudden death. In heart failure patients, the severity of heart failure, potential impact of the implantation procedure, and short-term prognosis from pump

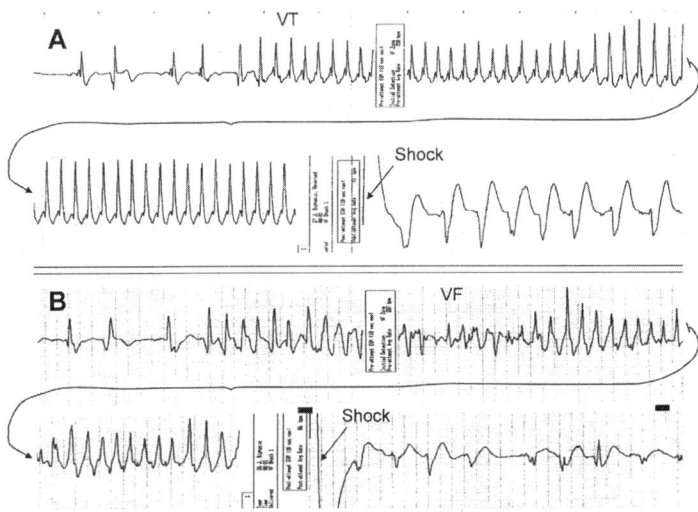

Figure 3–1. Tracings showing stored far-field electrograms from interrogation of the ICD in a patient with ischemic cardiomyopathy. Panel A was obtained after the patient reported an episode of syncope. Rapid monomorphic VT (average cycle length, 240 ms) was terminated by a single 27-J shock. Recurrent episodes of monomorphic VT were subsequently abolished by radiofrequency ablation. Three years later, the patient reported another episode of syncope. ICD interrogation (panel B) reveals atrial fibrillation (chronic) followed by abrupt onset spontaneous VF terminated by a single 26-J shock.

failure are also important considerations, influencing whether an ICD may be the best treatment for an individual patient.

Heart Failure Severity and Patient Selection

The severity of heart failure is an important consideration in assessing whether an ICD is warranted. Successful termination of VT or VF meaningfully extends survival when the patient has well-compensated heart failure and returns to the prearrhythmia functional state. Extension of survival is limited when deteriorating heart failure or associated complications lead to death from pump failure soon after an episode of VT (Figures 3–2 and 3–3).

Table 3-1

Randomized Trials of ICDs Versus Antiarrhythmic Drugs for Secondary Prevention of Sudden Death

	AVID[93]	CIDS[94]	CASH[76]
Target population	VT/VF survivors	VT/VF survivors	VF survivors
Treatment	ICD versus drug (amiodarone/sotalol)	ICD versus amiodarone	ICD vs. amiodarone vs. metoprolol[+]
Patients enrolled	1016	659	349
Arrhythmia qualifier	VF, syncopal VT, or poorly tolerated VT + LVEF <40%	VF, syncopal VT, VT >150 beats/min + LVEF <35%, syncope + inducible VT	VF requiring defibrillation
LVEF (%) qualifier	<40%	<35%	None
CHF (%)	42	~50	~27
NYHA II (%)	48	~38	57
NYHA III (%)	10	~10 (including IV)	16
NYHA IV (%)	Excluded	~10 (including III)	Excluded
Revascularization (%)	37	~30	~20
Mean LVEF (%)	31–32	33–34	>45
ACE inhibitors (%)	~66	Not reported	Not reported
Beta-blockers (%)	~42% ICD vs. 17% drug group	54% ICD vs. 23% amiodarone group	1/3 randomized to metoprolol alone
Outcome	Survival advantage in ICD group	Trend toward survival advantage in ICD group	Survival advantage in ICD group
Total mortality rate	11% ICD vs. 18% drug @ 1 year (RR 32%)	8.3%/yr ICD vs. 10.2%/yr amio (RR 19.7%, $P=0.14$)	12.1% ICD vs. 19.6% amio/metoprolol @ 2 years (RR 37%)
Sudden death rate	5% ICD vs. 11% drug (unadjusted)	3.0%/yr ICD vs. 4.5%/yr amio (RR 32%, $P=0.09$)	2% ICD vs. 11–12% amio/metoprolol
Comments	96% of drug group received empiric amiodarone; 40–45% had no CHF symptoms	Fewer patients had symptomatic CHF vs. AVID	[+]Propafenone arm stopped in 1992 due to excess mortality (all sudden deaths)

VF = ventricular fibrillation; VT = ventricular tachycardia; LVEF = left ventricular ejection fraction; CHF = congestive heart failure; NYHA = New York Heart Association Functional Class; RR = risk reduction.

Table 3–2

Indications for Implantable Defibrillators

Secondary Prevention after Cardiac Arrest
  Resuscitated from cardiac arrest not due to a clear reversible, correctable cause
  Controversial: cardiac arrest from a secondary cause in a patient with heart failure
Primary Prevention of Sudden Death
  Coronary artery disease + all of the following:
    LV ejection fraction ≤0.40
    Nonsustained VT
    Inducible VT at electrophysiology study
    Functional status better than New York Heart Association Class IV
  Unexplained syncope + heart failure
  Familial cardiomyopathy with high risk for sudden death
Indications Under Study
  All postinfarction patients with LV ejection fraction <0.30 (except Class IV)
  Postinfarction patients with depressed ventricular function and no inducible VT
  Nonischemic dilated cardiomyopathy

VT = ventricular tachycardia; LV = left ventricular.

Patients with severely decompensated heart failure are less likely to benefit from an ICD, and may suffer harm from the implantation and testing procedure (see below).

Although the ICD trials discussed (Tables 3–1 and 6–2) did not specifically enroll patients with heart failure, patients who have compensated heart failure (New York Heart Association functional Class I or II symptoms) fit the profile of patients enrolled in these trials (AVID, CASH, CIDS, MADIT, and MUSTT). The average left ventricular ejection fraction in these trials ranged from 0.26 to more than 0.4 and the majority of patients had some symptoms of cardiovascular limitation. Total mortality for patients in the AVID trial is similar to that reported for heart failure trials in patients with Class II-III symptoms (Figure 1–3). ICDs extend survival by preventing sudden arrhythmic death in these patients. Thus, mild to moderate heart failure is clearly not a contraindication to an ICD and high-risk patients are likely to benefit.

The risk-benefit balance of ICDs is more difficult to assess for patients with more advanced heart failure. The presence of Class

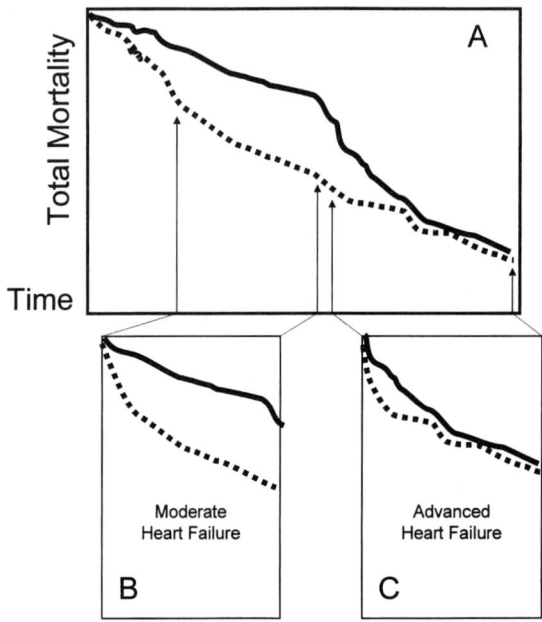

Figure 3–2. Theoretical survival curves for patients treated with a therapy that prevents sudden death due to arrhythmias, such as an ICD (solid line) compared to control. At the top (panel A) is a theoretical trial enrolling patients with mild heart failure followed until only 20% of the population remained, perhaps 15 to 20 years. Initially there is relatively little divergence of the curves because the risk of sudden death is low. However, with longer follow-up, the curves clearly diverge. Theoretical results for trials initiated in patients at later stages of heart failure are shown at the bottom in panels B and C. In panel B, a substantial mortality benefit is observed because the incidence of sudden deaths is low and there is a good chance for survival after resuscitation. In patients with advanced heart failure, progressive deaths from pump failure limit extension of survival.

IV symptoms excluded patients from the AVID, CASH, CIDS, MADIT, MADIT II, and MUSTT trials. In AVID, CASH, and CIDS, 90% of patients had functional Class I or II symptoms, and only 10% had functional Class III symptoms.[96] In a post hoc analysis of subgroups in the AVID trial, there was a survival benefit demonstrable for patients with ejection fractions between 0.20 and 0.34, but patients with worse left ventricular function (ejection fraction <0.20) did not have a statistically significant improvement in survival.[97] In a single-center retrospective study of

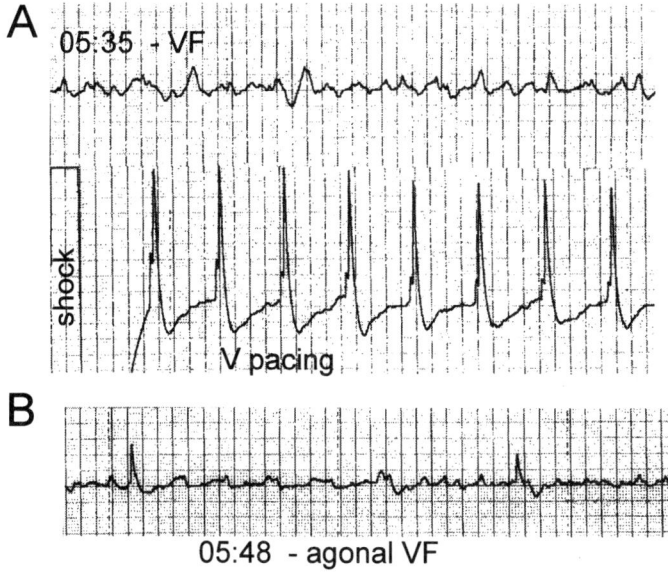

Figure 3–3. Selected tracings obtained from postmortem interrogation of an ICD after sudden death of a patient with ischemic cardiomyopathy and a history of sustained monomorphic VT who was awaiting cardiac transplantation. At 05:31 (not shown), a ventricular rate of 206 beats/min was detected and reverted to ventricular pacing after four consecutive 33-J shocks. The electrogram recorded 4 minutes later at 05:35 (panel A) shows a rapid rate consistent with VF. A single 33-J shock restores VVI pacing at 70 beats/min (electrogram 3). However, 13 minutes later (05:48), VF recurs (panel B). The low-amplitude electrograms suggest that fine VF, consistent with severe cardiac decompensation or metabolic deterioration, is present; device therapies failed to restore an effective circulation.

291 consecutive patients evaluated for cardiac transplantation, 12-month sudden death rates were lowest in patients treated with an ICD (9.2%), intermediate for patients who did not receive treatment for an arrhythmia (16%), and highest (35%) for patients treated with antiarrhythmic drugs, $P=0.004$.[98] Despite the lower incidence of sudden death, total mortality was similar among the three patient groups. In other studies, a greater benefit is observed in the sicker patients.[95] In a post hoc analysis of the CIDS trial, the

24 CLINICAL APPROACHES TO TACHYARRHYTHMIAS

study population was divided into quartiles of risk based on age, ejection fraction, and functional class. ICD therapy was associated with a 50% reduction in death in the highest risk quartile, but conferred no benefit in the three lower risk quartiles.[95] In the MADIT study, benefit appeared to be largely confined to patients with ejection fractions less than the median value of 26%.[99]

Thus, the benefit of ICD therapy as reflected by an extension of survival appears to follow a bell-shaped curve. Patients with mild heart failure generally have a lower risk of arrhythmia events and as a population receive less benefit during initial follow-up. With increasing severity of heart failure, the incidence of arrhythmic events (VT and VF) increases such that the benefit of the ICD increases, until mortality from pump failure increases to the extent that effective arrhythmia termination minimally extends survival (Figure 3-2).[100] In some cases, heart failure symptoms become intolerable and patients seek to have the tachyarrhythmia therapies of the device turned off to allow a more natural death. Extrapolating data from trials to an individual patient is often difficult. The patient's age also influences the likely benefit, with very high 1-year mortality of approximately 50% despite an ICD for patients older than 85 years of age observed in one preliminary report.[101]

In general, patients with compensated heart failure are candidates for ICD implantation when they have an indication for an ICD. Some patients with decompensated heart failure should not receive an ICD, even though the risk of ventricular arrhythmias is high. When antiarrhythmic therapy is required, amiodarone may be a better option. However, it should be remembered that some patients with Class IV symptoms at one point in time survive for years after resuscitation from a cardiac arrhythmia.[102]

The possibility for cardiac transplantation also impacts on the potential benefit of an ICD. Most patients who are accepted onto elective transplantation waiting lists are sufficiently compensated to wait at home for a donor heart to become available. Sudden death is a significant risk for these patients. Of 434 patients accepted onto the elective transplantation list between 1984 and 1997 at one center, 25% received a donor heart, 26% of patients died, and 72% of these deaths were sudden.[58] Even for patients who have very poor functional capacity, a dramatic extension of survival occurs when successful defibrillation allows a patient to receive a transplant. Protection from sudden arrhythmic death with an ICD allows some patients with advanced heart failure to await cardiac transplantation at home, avoiding or delaying in-patient waiting until hemodynamic deterioration necessitates inotropic support. Implantation of an ICD is a reasonable consideration even though progressive hemodynamic deterioration is anticipated.[58,98,103]

Bradycardia Pacing with ICDs

All ICDs incorporate pacing for bradycardia. Dual chamber (AV) pacing, activity responsiveness, and mode switching for atrial arrhythmias are available. Approximately 50% of patients who require ICD therapy have indications for or subsequently evolve the need for permanent pacing for bradyarrhythmia.[104] Use of the ICD for bradycardia pacing is preferable to placement of a separate pacemaker, thereby avoiding adverse interactions between the devices and minimizing the number of leads implanted. If sinus rhythm, rather than atrial fibrillation, is present, maintenance of AV synchrony is generally preferred (Chapter 8). This is achieved with a dual chamber defibrillator that requires placement of an atrial lead as well as the ventricular lead.

Although AV pacing is generally preferred to ventricular pacing alone, the consequences of AV pacing warrant careful consideration due to the potential for adverse hemodynamic effects of right ventricular apical pacing. As discussed in Chapter 8, right ventricular apical pacing, which produces QRS prolongation similar to left bundle branch block, is associated with worse ventricular performance than ventricular activation over the normal His-Purkinje system, which produces a shorter QRS duration.[105-107] It appears desirable to avoid right ventricular apical pacing when there is normal ventricular activation (i.e., narrow QRS duration). Optimal pacing operation in current dual chamber ICD systems necessitates short pacemaker AV intervals, such that ventricular pacing usually occurs in the DDD mode, even when AV conduction is intact. In some patients, backup VVI pacing below the intrinsic heart rate, which results in supraventricular conduction and rare ventricular pacing, might be preferable to chronic RV apical pacing in the DDD mode. The implementation of left ventricular pacing (cardiac resynchronization) may obviate this concern, but further investigation is required.

Perioperative Considerations: Minimizing Risks of ICD Implantation

Up to 50% of patients who receive an ICD will experience an adverse effect at some time.[108] Complications of implantation include pneumothorax or hemothorax, ventricular perforation, pocket infections or fluid collections, lead dislodgment, and venous thrombosis and embolism. The implantation procedure usually includes initiation of VF and testing of defibrillation from the ICD to make certain that the lead configuration and energy available will effectively defibrillate. Induced VF is associated with mild, transient ventricular dysfunction, which is well tolerated in the majority of patients.[109] In patients with advanced heart failure, defibrillation threshold testing occasionally precipitates a hemodynamic deterioration (Figure 3–4). In one series, 3 of 59 patients (5%) who were being evaluated for cardiac transplantation developed electromechanical dissociation after successful defibrillation.[98] In decompensated patients, ICD implantation should be deferred until medical therapy has been optimized and heart failure improved. In general, the mortality from defibrillation implantation is less than 1%, but this risk has not been specifically assessed in heart failure populations.

Many patients with heart failure have atrial fibrillation or other indications for chronic anticoagulation with warfarin. Device pocket hematomas are an important early problem for these patients. In one study, pocket hematomas developed in 22% of patients who received therapy with heparin starting 6 hours after pacemaker or ICD implantation, in 17% of patients who received heparin starting 24 hours after implantation, and in 1% to 2% of patients who did not receive anticoagulation or in whom therapy with warfarin was initiated without heparin therapy.[110] Pocket hematomas cause pain, immobility, can delay hospital discharge

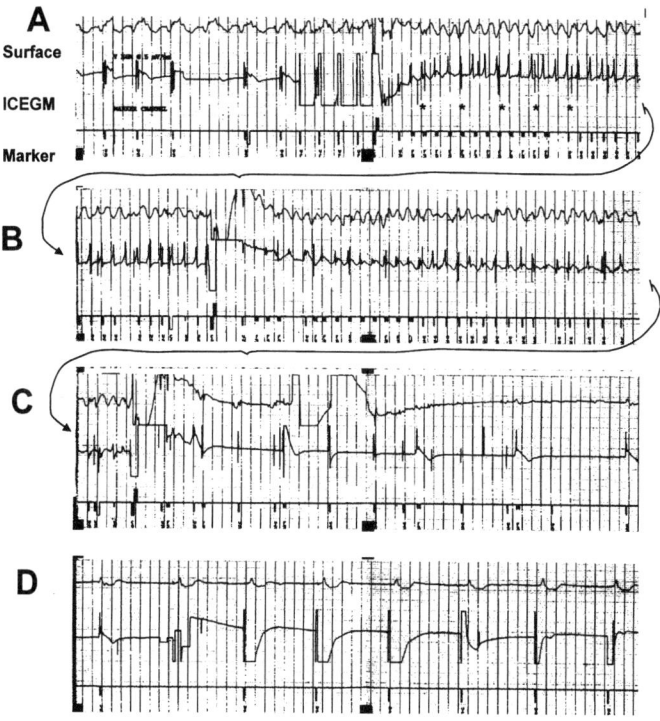

Figure 3–4. These tracings were obtained during defibrillation testing at the time of ICD implantation in a 44-year-old male with severe non-ischemic dilated cardiomyopathy due to cardiac sarcoidosis. A separate DDDR pacing system was previously implanted due to complete heart block. The tracings (panels A–D) are continuous. From the top of each tracing are the surface ECG, intracardiac electrogram recorded from the ICD lead, and the marker channel that specifies the ICD classification of sensed events and responses. In panel A, VF is intentionally initiated by a T-wave shock. Note ventricular pacing spikes (*) from the separate pacing system continue during VF. A 20-J shock fails to terminate VF (B) followed by a 30-J shock that terminates VF (C). After VF termination, ventricular pacing at maximum output (7.5 V/1.5 ms) fails to capture. The ineffectual pacing stimuli from the separate pacemaker are sensed by the ICD and inhibit bradycardia pacing by the ICD. Agonal ventricular escape rhythm (arrows) develops. Chest fluoroscopy revealed absent cardiac motion. Cardiopulmonary resuscitation was initiated. After approximately 10 minutes, ventricular capture was restored (D). Hemodynamic recovery required inotropic support and the patient remained hospitalized until cardiac transplantation.

and patient recovery, and may increase the risk of infection. The timing and method of reinstitution of anticoagulation must be carefully considered on an individual basis for patients with a chronic indication for anticoagulation. Infection occurs in fewer than 1% of devices with completely transvenous lead systems, but is a major problem when it occurs.[111,112] Diabetics are more susceptible. Active infection is a contraindication to device implantation.

Continuing Care

Patients with ICDs should be followed in a specialized clinic. Routine device interrogations assessing sensing and pacing function, remaining battery life, and arrhythmias detected by the ICD are generally performed every 3 to 4 months.

Up to 40% of patients receive inappropriate therapies from the ICD at some point during follow-up (Figure 3–5). Heart rate is the major criterion for arrhythmia detection. A rate exceeding the programmed detection threshold will trigger therapy with either antitachycardia pacing (ATP) or high-voltage shocks. Thus, sinus tachycardia or a rapid supraventricular tachycardia can lead to painful shocks. Inappropriate therapy, as for rapid atrial fibrillation or flutter, can often be recognized and managed with reprogramming of the ICD. Occasionally, inappropriate therapy is due to oversensing of diaphragmatic activity or T-waves. Electrical noise indicating a lead fracture or loose connection of the lead in the pulse generator header can also cause inappropriate shocks.

Following the first symptomatic therapy from the ICD after implantation, patient assessment with interrogation of the device is usually warranted to confirm appropriate function of the ICD and to assess the possibility that therapy was inappropriate, triggered by a supraventricular arrhythmia (see Figure 3–5). If the patient receives more than one shock in a short period of time or has symptoms of arrhythmia or a change in symptoms that persists following an ICD shock, urgent evaluation is required. Failure of ICD therapy to terminate the arrhythmia, persistence of a VT at a rate that is slower than the programmed detection criteria, or persistence of a supraventricular arrhythmia, such as atrial fibrilla-

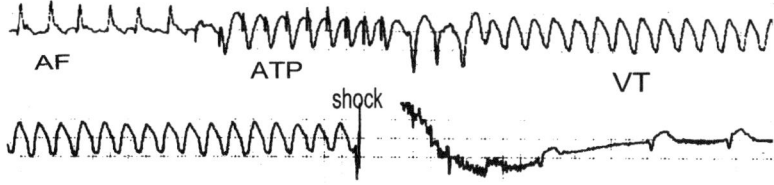

Figure 3–5. A single ECG lead monitor tracing from a patient with an ICD who was recovering from recent coronary artery surgery. Rapid atrial fibrillation occurred, and exceeded the rate detection criteria for VT. The ICD applies a burst of rapid antitachycardia pacing (ATP), which initiates VT. The rapid VT elicits a high-voltage shock from the ICD, terminating both the VT and atrial fibrillation. Unfortunately, atrial fibrillation recurred such that this sequence of events occurred several times before the ICD was temporarily inactivated by application of a magnet and additional therapy to reduce the rate of atrial fibrillation was administered.

tion, are possible causes. Repeated episodes of VT or VF are a marker for greater mortality, are often associated with hemodynamic deterioration, and warrant urgent assessment.[113-115] Myocardial ischemia, electrolyte disturbances, and intercurrent illness are important potential causes of arrhythmia exacerbations that should be considered. Patients who have infrequent episodes of VT usually do not require immediate evaluation when symptoms indicate that another episode of tachycardia has been terminated by the ICD, provided that the episode is similar to previous episodes.

ICDs terminate VT by either antitachycardia pacing or delivering a high-voltage shock (Figure 3–1). Antitachycardia pacing is painless and well tolerated; some patients experience palpitations, but many are unaware that they have received a therapy. Shocks for cardioversion or defibrillation are painful and usually not well tolerated. Patients who receive frequent, symptomatic ICD therapies usually require additional treatment to prevent arrhythmia recurrences, either antiarrhythmic drug therapy or catheter ablation.

Occasionally, it is necessary to temporarily disable an ICD to prevent incessant shocks or antitachycardia pacing such as may be triggered by an "electrical storm" of recurrent VT or atrial fibrillation with a rapid ventricular response in a patient in the intensive care unit (Figure 3–5).[115] Application of a magnet over the ICD pulse generator suspends arrhythmia detection as long as the magnet is in place, allowing time for implementation of other therapy. While the magnet is in place, the patient must be closely monitored and external cardioversion used as appropriate to treat arrhythmias.

Antiarrhythmic Drug Interactions with ICDs

Many patients with ICDs require antiarrhythmic drug therapy to control supraventricular arrhythmias (most commonly atrial fibrillation and flutter) or reduce episodes of VT. In the presence of an ICD, the potential for fatal drug-induced proarrhythmia is low. The ICD will terminate torsades de pointes and provide pacing for bradyarrhythmias. Antiarrhythmic drugs can impede effective ICD termination of arrhythmias and should be used cautiously.

Some antiarrhythmic drugs increase the current required for defibrillation. At the time of ICD implantation, defibrillation testing is performed by inducing VF and observing that an ICD shock below the maximum energy available from the ICD will terminate fibrillation. Most ICDs are capable of providing a 28- to 35-joule shock. A 10-joule safety margin is recommended and confirmed by demonstrating that VF is terminated by a shock 10 joules below the maximum energy available from the ICD. Amiodarone therapy typically increases the energy required for defibrillation. If the defibrillation threshold is close to the maximal energy of the ICD, antiarrhythmic drug therapy may increase it such that maximal energy shocks from the ICD are no longer effective. Other antiarrhythmic drugs may also increase the defibrillation threshold, although less predictably than amiodarone, and data are conflicting. Class III antiarrhythmic drugs that block potassium channels, sotalol and dofetilide, may decrease the defibrillation threshold. In general, repeat defibrillation testing is warranted when chronic therapy with an antiarrhythmic drug is administered, with the possible exceptions of beta-blockers, sotalol, and dofetilide.

Antiarrhythmic drug therapy often slows a VT. If the tachycardia rate falls below the programmed detection rate, the arrhythmia will not be recognized or treated by the ICD. This problem can be solved by reducing the programmed VT detection rate, but sinus tachycardia or atrial arrhythmias will then be more likely to exceed the detection rate, eliciting inappropriate therapy. Antiarrhythmic drug therapy can alter the amplitude of sensed endocardial electrograms and/or pacing thresholds, but this problem is uncommon.

Psychological Support

The presence of an ICD "safety net" is greatly reassuring for most patients. Those who have experienced repeated, painful ICD shocks, however, often live in fear of an arrhythmia recurrence.[116-120] Some patients needlessly restrict activities and suffer significant depression and anxiety. Patient support groups and counseling are often beneficial. Some patients require therapy with anxiolytics and antidepressant medications.

Summary

ICDs provide effective and reliable treatment of sustained VT and fibrillation and can be expected to decrease the risk of arrhythmic death in patients with heart failure. Whether this benefit translates to an overall improvement in survival depends on the severity of pump dysfunction. Appropriate patient selection for ICDs is an important aspect of arrhythmia management. Future devices will incorporate features that hope to reduce atrial arrhythmias, improve ventricular function, and monitor hemodynamics, as well as prevent sudden arrhythmic death.

4

The Cardiac Arrest Survivor

At the time of referral to a tertiary center, 11% of patients have already been resuscitated from a cardiac arrest and most will have an ICD already implanted.[14] Heart failure patients who are resuscitated from a cardiac arrest generally fit one of three different clinical profiles. The first are those patients with well-compensated heart failure and a primary arrhythmic event. If they are promptly resuscitated, they return to the "prearrest" state with preserved functional capacity. These patients resemble those addressed in the secondary prevention trial of ICDs (AVID, CASH, CIDS) (Chapter 3, Table 3–1); an ICD offers the best protection from sudden death.[76,93–95] At the other end of the clinical spectrum are those patients who have advanced Class IV heart failure in whom VT or VF occurs as a terminal or preterminal event. Termination of VT or VF, whether by paramedical personnel or an ICD, minimally extends life and may not be consonant with the patient's wishes and best interest. Between these two extremes are patients in whom cardiac arrest occurs as their heart failure status is beginning to deteriorate. Following resuscitation from the arrest, heart failure is a bit worse, and may improve further, but the patient is gradually deteriorating with a clinical course punctuated by episodes of ventricular arrhythmia (Figure 4–1).

Initial Patient Evaluation

Following resuscitation from sustained VT or VF, correctable precipitating factors, such as electrolyte abnormalities and acute myocardial infarction or ischemia, should be sought and addressed (Table 4–1, Figure 4–2). Hemodynamic function is often worse after the arrest; adjustment of medical therapy for heart failure is often required. Hemodynamic deterioration may be due to the hemodynamic insult from the arrest or from the event that precipitated

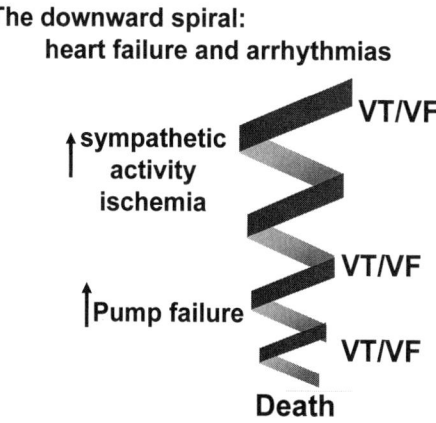

Figure 4–1. The downward spiral of heart failure. Sustained ventricular arrhythmias are often followed by transient exacerbations of heart failure that become more severe as heart failure deteriorates. Fluctuating renal perfusion, electrolyte disturbances, and drug levels likely contribute to instability.

the arrest, such as myocardial infarction or ischemia, pulmonary embolism, or deteriorating renal function with hyperkalemia (Figure 4–3). In one series, cardiac arrest was attributed to a secondary cause in 42% of patients with a history of chronic heart failure.[13]

Ventricular fibrillation is most commonly encountered at the time of the arrest and is often initiated by VT.[14,121] Electrophysiologic study can be used to assess the presence of inducible arrhythmias, but is not required for most patients. Electrophysiologic testing does allow assessment of the presence of scar-related reentrant VT or bundle branch reentry, but therapy with an ICD is reasonable for many of these patients regardless of the outcome of electrophysiologic testing (see below). Electrophysiologic study should be performed if a supraventricular arrhythmia is suspected as the precipitating cause.[122,123] Although precipitating supraventricular arrhythmias are infrequent, occurring in fewer than 6% of cardiac arrests, they are an important consideration. Implantation of an ICD without treating the supraventricular arrhythmia will likely be followed by inappropriate shocks when supraventricular arrhythmias recur.

Table 4–1
Causes and Precipitating Factors for Cardiac Arrest in Heart Failure

Primary Cardiac Arrest
  monomorphic ventricular tachycardia
  polymorphic ventricular tachycardia
  atrioventricular block
  sinus arrest

Secondary Cardiac Arrest/Precipitating Causes
  myocardial ischemia or infarction
  pulmonary embolism
  stroke
  rapid supraventricular tachycardia
  QT prolongation with torsades de pointes
  respiratory arrest/pulmonary edema followed by cardiac arrest
  potassium: hyperkalemia or hypokalemia
  calcium: hypocalcemia or hypercalcemia
  hypoglycemia
  exsanguination: ruptured aortic aneurysm

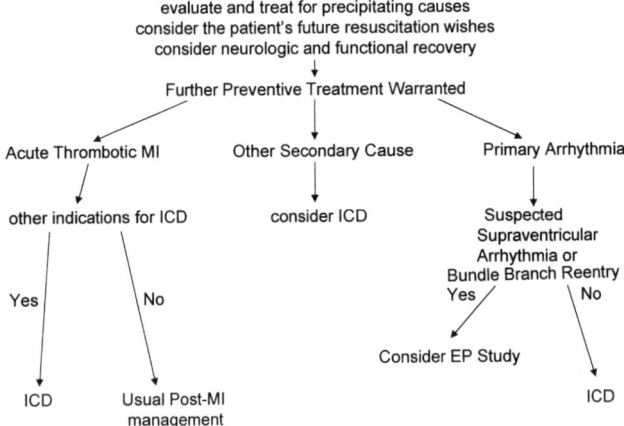

Figure 4–2. Flow diagram for the evaluation and management of patients with heart failure who are resuscitated from a cardiac arrest. ICD = implantable cardioverter-defibrillator; MI = myocardial infarction.

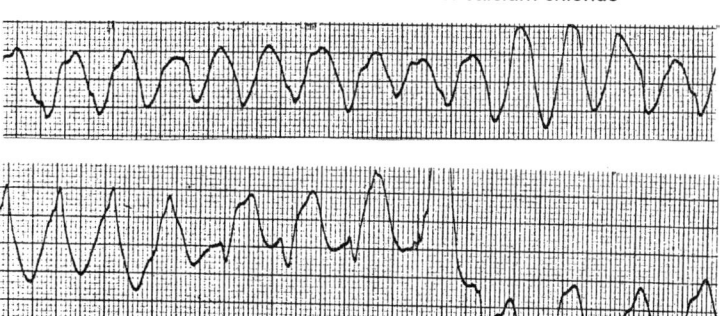

Figure 4–3. Sinusoidal VT due to hyperkalemia. Intravenous administration of calcium chloride results in gradual narrowing of the QRS complex and subsequent return of sinus rhythm (not shown).

Primary Cardiac Arrest

Patients resuscitated from VT or VF that is not due to a secondary cause have a high risk of recurrent arrhythmia, approximately 20% per year, even if antiarrhythmic drug therapy is administered.[124,125] The likelihood of recurrent arrhythmia increases with severity of ventricular dysfunction.[124] Patients who present with VT are more likely to have recurrences compared to those who present with VF.[124,126,127]

ICDs are the major first-line therapy for cardiac arrest survivors (Table 3–1).[76,93–96] Meta-analysis of the secondary prevention trials AVID, CIDS, and CASH suggest a 28% reduction in total mortality that is attributable to a 50% reduction in sudden death.[96] A greater benefit was observed in patients with left ventricular ejection fraction below 0.35 than in those with better ventricular function. It is important to recognize that these trials did not specifically target heart failure populations, and Class IV patients were excluded. As discussed in Chapter 3, the long-term benefit is likely to be less in patients with advanced heart failure, and the severity of the patient's heart failure and other comorbidities should be considered in selecting therapy. An ICD may not be the best option for a patient with end-stage heart failure and no option for cardiac transplantation. Amiodarone is an alternative therapy for patients in whom an ICD is deemed not to be a reasonable option.

Secondary Cardiac Arrest

Patients who survive a cardiac arrest that is due to a presumed "secondary" cause have a high risk for sudden death even if the precipitating cause is recognized and treatment is instituted.[13,128–131] Causes of 22 secondary cardiac arrests in one series of patients with advanced heart failure included decompensated heart failure with pulmonary edema precipitating VF (9 patients) or a bradyarrhythmia (2 patients), torsades de pointes due to a drug (10 patients), and monomorphic VT precipitated by hypokalemia (1 patient).[13] Within 1 year, 32% of these patients died suddenly. In the AVID registry, 88 patients who had a left ventricular ejection fraction <0.35 and VT or VF attributed to a correctable cause had a 2-year total mortality of 29%.[128] The majority had coronary artery disease and many were treated with revascularization. Whether death was sudden or due to an arrhythmia is, however, not known. A secondary arrest may be a marker of electrical instability that persists even after treatment of the precipitating factor. Whether implantable defibrillators reduce sudden death in this population is not yet known, but implantation of an ICD is a reasonable consideration for many of these patients.

Summary

ICDs are the first-line therapy for preventing death from ventricular arrhythmias in patients who have been resuscitated from a cardiac arrest. Neurological and cardiac functional recovery are major factors that determine whether an ICD is appropriate in this patient population. Even when a secondary precipitating cause is identified, such as hypokalemia, the risk of death remains high; an ICD is often a reasonable consideration.

5

Sustained Ventricular Tachycardia

Ventricular tachycardia is designated sustained if it requires electrical cardioversion or administration of an antiarrhythmic drug for termination, or if it causes severe symptoms, such as syncope, before terminating. VTs are further classified based on the QRS configuration (Figure 5–1). Monomorphic VTs have the same QRS complex from beat to beat, indicating that the ventricles are repetitively depolarized with the same activation sequence. A structural abnormality supporting reentry or an arrhythmia focus is present. Polymorphic VTs have a changing QRS configuration from beat to beat, indicating a continually changing ventricular activation sequence. A structural focus causing the arrhythmia may be present but is not required.

Monomorphic Ventricular Tachycardia

Rapid VT often precipitates hemodynamic collapse followed by VF. If the patient is stable in VT, it is important to obtain a 12-lead electrocardiogram. The major diagnostic consideration is to distinguish VT from supraventricular tachycardia with bundle branch block aberrancy. Atrioventricular dissociation is strong evidence for VT. Specific QRS morphology criteria that have been developed for distinguishing VT from supraventricular tachycardia are not as reliable when severe ventricular enlargement and advanced heart failure are present (see Figure 9–2 below).[132–135] When the diagnosis is not certain, an electrophysiology study (EPS) is often helpful in making this important distinction.

Monomorphic VT is usually due to reentry through a region of ventricular scar (Figure 5–2). An old myocardial infarction is the most common cause. Areas of large ventricular scars also occur in nonischemic cardiomyopathies, but are much less common. Hence, monomorphic VT is more common in patients with prior infarction as compared to patients with nonischemic car-

38 CLINICAL APPROACHES TO TACHYARRHYTHMIAS

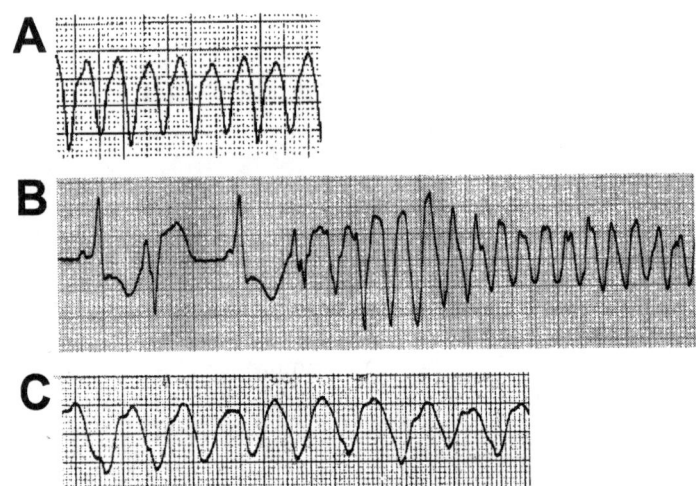

Figure 5–1. Types of ventricular tachycardia: monomorphic VT in panel A, polymorphic VT in panel B, sinusoidal VT due to hyperkalemia in panel C.

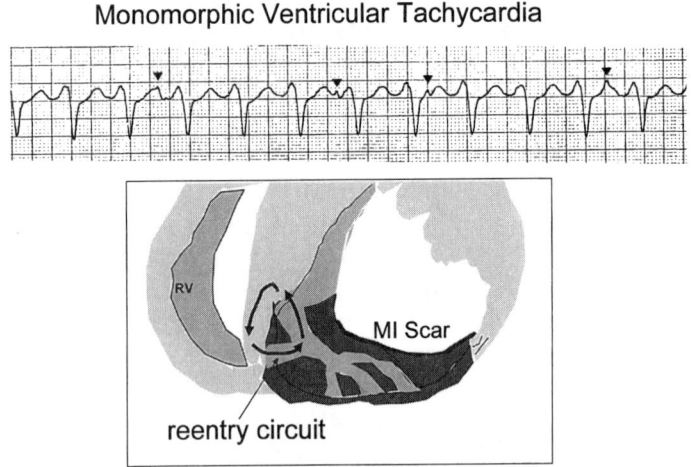

Figure 5–2. Sustained monomorphic VT due to reentry in an area of prior myocardial infarction. The schematic of the left ventricle at the bottom shows an inferior wall infarct with dense areas of fibrosis (dark areas) and surviving myocyte bundles (gray) that form channels through the infarct supporting a reentry circuit (arrows).

diomyopathies. In patients with nonischemic cardiomyopathies, large areas of scar causing monomorphic VT are most likely in sarcoidosis, arrhythmogenic right ventricular dysplasia, and Chagas' disease, or when a coronary embolism from a left atrial or ventricular thrombus causes a myocardial infarction.

The QRS morphology of monomorphic VT often suggests the origin and sometimes the etiology of the VT. VTs that have a left bundle branch block configuration in V_1 usually originate in the interventricular septum or in the right ventricle. Arrhythmogenic right ventricular dysplasia, bundle branch reentry (see below), and a left ventricular septal area of scar are possible causes.

Bundle Branch Reentry

Slowed conduction through the His-Purkinje system, often associated with severe ventricular dysfunction, predisposes to this uncommon type of VT.[22,136] The reentry excitation wavefront propagates down the right bundle branch, through the interventricular septum, and then up the left bundle branch to complete the circuit. The tachycardia then has a left bundle branch block-like configuration (Figure 5–3). Less commonly, the circuit revolves in the opposite direction, giving rise to VT with a right bundle branch block configuration in lead V_1. Bundle branch reentry does not require the presence of ventricular scar. It should be particularly suspected in patients with monomorphic VT and non-ischemic dilated cardiomyopathy, valvular heart disease, or cardiomyopathy associated with muscular dystrophy. It causes 20% to 30% of sustained monomorphic VTs in patients with nonischemic dilated cardiomyopathy and fewer than 5% of monomorphic VTs in patients with prior infarction.[22,136] Most patients have intraventricular conduction delay evident during the sinus rhythm. The QRS morphology of the VT can resemble that of the interventricular conduction delay observed during sinus rhythm, falsely suggesting supraventricular tachycardia with aberrant conduction.[135] The VT is often rapid, typically 215 beats/min, leading to hemodynamic collapse and presenting with cardiac arrest.

Although bundle branch reentry is relatively easily cured by catheter ablation of the right bundle branch (Figure 5–3, panel B),

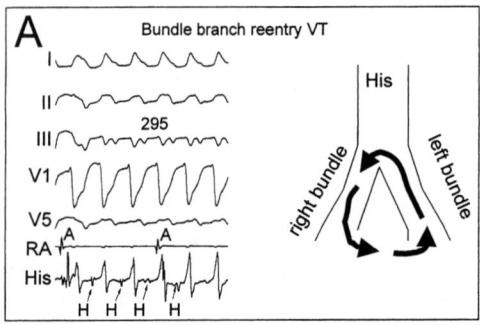
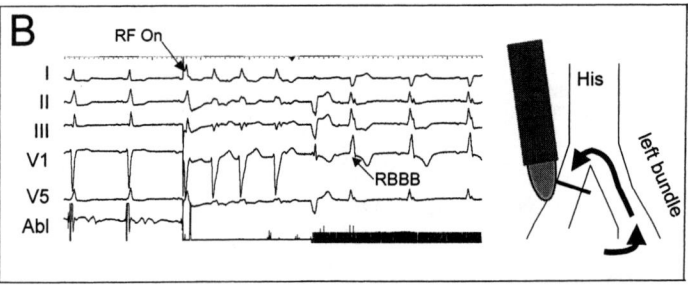

Figure 5–3. Bundle branch reentry tachycardia. In panel A, tachycardia recorded during EP study shows dissociated atrial activity (A deflections in the right atrial tracing [HRA]), with His bundle deflections before every QRS. In panel B, radiofrequency catheter ablation of the right bundle produces right bundle branch block and effectively prevents further bundle branch reentry tachycardia as illustrated in the schematic at the right.

some patients have other VTs inducible as well, and 20% to 30% of patients will require implantation of a permanent pacemaker after ablation. Implantation of an ICD that offers backup bradycardia pacing is also a reasonable first option, with catheter ablation reserved for patients who experience recurrent arrhythmias.

Arrhythmogenic Right Ventricular Cardiomyopathy

Arrhythmogenic right ventricular cardiomyopathy (also known as arrhythmogenic right ventricular dysplasia) is an important diagnostic concern for patients with VTs that have a left bundle branch block-like configuration in V_1.[24–28] Portions of the right ventricle are replaced with fibrous and fatty tissue, causing reentry circuits. The left ventricle is involved in over 30% of cases and left ventricular failure can occur and dominate the clinical presentation.[25,137] This disease appears to have a genetic basis, and a family history of sudden death or VT can be found in approximately 40% of patients. The sinus rhythm electrocardiogram often shows T-wave inversion in the anterior precordial leads and QRS duration exceeding 110 ms in V_2.[27] Magnetic resonance imaging usually identifies intramural areas of fatty infiltrate in the right ventricular wall, but distinguishing areas that are clearly abnormal from areas of normal epicardial fat is often difficult. Echocardiography or contrast ventriculography reveals an enlarged right ventricle or aneurysm formation in some cases, but is often interpreted as normal. At EPS, sustained monomorphic VT is usually inducible if it has occurred spontaneously. Mapping of the right ventricle identifies areas of abnormal, low-amplitude electrograms similar to those observed for scar-related VTs after myocardial infarction.[23] The presence of multiple morphologies of inducible VT and areas of low-amplitude electrograms distinguishes arrhythmogenic right ventricular dysplasia from idiopathic right VT (see below).

Recurrent episodes of VT are common and are often provoked by exercise. Patients with left ventricular involvement have a worse prognosis than those with involvement limited to the right ventricle and sometimes require cardiac transplantation for progressive heart failure.

Idiopathic Ventricular Tachycardia Causing Tachycardia-Induced Heart Failure

Idiopathic VTs refer to a group of monomorphic VTs that typically occur in patients who do not have structural heart disease. In rare cases, an incessant idiopathic VT will lead to tachycardia-induced heart failure that resolves when the arrhythmia is controlled.[138–141] The most common type of idiopathic VT originates from a focus in the right ventricular outflow tract.[142,143] The tachycardia has a left bundle branch block-like configuration with an axis that is directed inferiorly, giving rise to tall positive R-waves in leads II, III, and aVF. Arrhythmogenic right ventricular dysplasia can produce tachycardia with a similar morphology and is the major diagnostic concern.

When incessant tachycardia is the cause of heart failure and depressed ventricular function, abolition of the VT by catheter ablation or antiarrhythmic drug therapy is followed by gradual recovery of ventricular function that may continue to improve over the next year. Implantation of an ICD is usually not warranted.

Long-Term Therapy for Sustained Monomorphic VT

Following restoration of sinus rhythm, potential precipitating and aggravating factors should be sought and corrected. However, it should be recognized that sustained monomorphic VT is associated with an underlying structural abnormality in the vast majority of cases and that the risk of recurrence is high regardless of antiarrhythmic drug therapy or correction of myocardial ischemia or other potential aggravating factors. When monomorphic VT occurs with elevated serum cardiac enzymes indicating infarction, the risk of recurrent VT remains high despite treatment for ischemia.[144] When VT is related to an area of scar or bundle branch reentry, the risk of recurrence exceeds 40%.

This type of VT is inducible in the electrophysiology laboratory in >90% of patients, allowing electrophysiologic testing to be used for confirmation of the diagnosis and guiding ablation therapy, if needed. If the wide QRS presenting arrhythmia might be supraventricular tachycardia with aberrant conduction, an EPS should be performed to clarify the diagnosis. In over 90% of cases, a regular, wide QRS tachycardia in a patient with a history of prior myocardial infarction is VT rather than supraventricular tachycardia with aberrancy, even if the arrhythmia is hemodynamically tolerated.

If VT is incessant, it should be suppressed with antiarrhythmic drug therapy or catheter ablation.[145] The possibility of idiopathic VT causing tachycardia-induced cardiomyopathy should be considered.

Implantation of an ICD is recommended for patients with VT that causes hemodynamic compromise, provided that the patient is a candidate for an ICD. VT that is hemodynamically tolerated is associated with a lower risk of sudden death than VT that presents with syncope or cardiac arrest. In patients with poor ventricular function, however, a relatively high mortality rate has been observed in retrospective analyses.[146,147] In patients with depressed ventricular function, an ICD is a reasonable option even if VT is hemodynamically tolerated. The device can often terminate the arrhythmia by antitachycardia pacing. If VT recurs causing symptomatic ICD therapies, the addition of antiarrhythmic drugs or catheter ablation can be considered at that time.

Polymorphic Ventricular Tachycardia

Polymorphic VT (Figure 5–1, panel B) has a continually changing QRS complex. It is often caused by a potentially reversible condition. Acute myocardial ischemia or infarction is a common cause of polymorphic VT, and assessment for ischemia and infarction are warranted. Torsades de pointes is the other major form of polymorphic VT. Less commonly, polymorphic VT occurs associated with cardiomyopathy or prior infarction without clear precipitating triggers.

Torsades de Pointes

Polymorphic VT associated with QT interval prolongation is referred to as torsades de pointes (Figure 5–4).[148] Any cause of QT interval prolongation can cause torsades de pointes.[15,149–151] Electrophysiologic changes in chronic heart failure may increase susceptibility to torsades de pointes (Chapter 1). Hypokalemia, bradycardia, drugs such as sotalol, dofetilide, ibutilide, quinidine, n-acetylprocainamide, haloperidol, and erythromycin are relatively common causes. A more extensive list is available at the *www.QTdrugs.org* website maintained by Georgetown University.

Torsades de pointes is often "bradycardia-dependent" or "pause-dependent," with a characteristic initiating sequence (Fig-

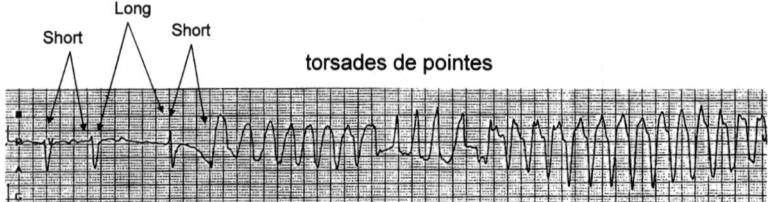

Figure 5–4. The polymorphic VT torsades de pointes with a typical short–long–short initiating sequence of R-R intervals is shown. The underlying rhythm is atrial flutter. This arrhythmia was due to accumulation of n-acetylprocainamide (NAPA) in a patient with renal failure who was receiving procainamide.

ure 5–4). A sudden increase in R-R interval, as may occur following a premature beat, creates a pause. The QT interval of the beat terminating the pause is prolonged. The first beat of the tachycardia interrupts the T-wave of that beat. Interventions that increase heart rate and shorten refractoriness are protective. Emergent treatment to prevent recurrent episodes is intravenous administration of 1 to 2 gm of magnesium sulfate. If episodes continue, therapy directed at accelerating the heart rate with intravenous administration of isoproterenol and/or transvenous pacing is warranted.

Patients who have had torsades de pointes should avoid all drugs that prolong the QT interval. Although amiodarone prolongs the QT interval, it rarely causes torsades de pointes, possibly because it also blocks ionic currents that also cause the arrhythmia. However, patients with heart failure are particularly susceptible to torsades de pointes and therapy with amiodarone is not protective.[2,8] Treatment with an ICD is a reasonable consideration. ICDs also provide pacing to prevent bradycardia and suppress pauses following premature beats that may help prevent polymorphic VT.[152]

6

Primary Prevention of Arrhythmic Sudden Death:

Nonsustained Ventricular Tachycardia and Other Potential Markers of Risk

While appropriate treatment of patients who have suffered a sustained ventricular arrhythmia can improve survival (secondary prevention), the majority of patients do not survive their first cardiac arrest. Identifying patients at risk for a cardiac arrest prior to its occurrence (primary prevention) is the focus of much research. For a marker of risk to be useful clinically requires demonstration that: (1) the marker identifies a high-risk group, and (2) specific therapy directed at the high-risk group improves survival. Several noninvasive markers of potential electrical instability, such as ambient ventricular ectopy, including nonsustained VT, heart rate variability, and measures of repolarization abnormality, have a physiological basis for predicting arrhythmia risk (Table 6–1). However, in most cases, the prevalence of abnormal markers increases in parallel with the severity of heart failure and, disappointingly, these markers have not been found to be specific for arrhythmia risk.

Depressed Left Ventricular Function

The severity of heart failure and systolic dysfunction is related to the risk of sudden death (Figure 1–3). The MADIT II trial randomized 1232 patients with coronary artery disease and a left ventricular ejection fraction <0.30 to receive an ICD or to no specific antiarrhythmic therapy, with three out of every five patients directed to the ICD arm. Class IV patients were excluded; 56% of patients had functional Class II or III symptoms. The trial was stopped in November 2001 after examination of the data revealed a significantly better survival for patients treated with an ICD.[153] If scrutiny of the data and other ongoing trials confirm this report, it will be reasonable to consider an ICD for this group of patients.

Table 6–1
Markers of Sudden Death Risk

Nonsustained VT
    Related to mortality and sudden death risk
    Suppression with amiodarone does not substantially reduce risk
    In patients with coronary artery disease programmed stimulation can be used to further define risk

Invasive Electrophysiologic Testing for Inducible VT
    Useful in patients with prior infarction; patients with inducible VT benefit from an ICD
    Not useful for risk stratification in patients with nonischemic cardiomyopathy; but can be considered if symptoms suggest an arrhythmia or if a specific cardiomyopathy associated with scar-related VT is suspected (e.g., arrhythmogenic right ventricular dysplasia, cardiac involvement with sarcoidosis)

AV Block
    Related to sudden death risk in nonischemic cardiomyopathy in one study

Signal-Averaged Electrocardiogram
    Abnormal test is related to inducible VT and sudden death risk in patients with prior myocardial infarction
    Insufficient evidence to warrant antiarrhythmic treatment based on this test alone

Heart Rate Variability
    Depressed heart rate variability is associated with increased mortality and increased sudden death risk in some studies
    Insufficient evidence to warrant antiarrhythmic treatment based on this test alone

QT Interval Dispersion
    Unreliable

Beat-to-Beat QT Dynamicity
    Investigational

T-Wave Alternans
    Related to arrhythmia risk
    Insufficient evidence to warrant antiarrhythmic treatment based on this test alone

VT = ventricular tachycardia; ICD = implantable cardioverter-defibrillator.

Nonsustained Ventricular Tachycardia and Ventricular Ectopic Activity

Ventricular ectopic activity and nonsustained VT of three or more consecutive beats (Figure 6–1) are common in heart failure patients; 34% to 79% of patients have one or more runs of nonsustained VT on 24-hour ambulatory recordings.[62,154,155] In the Prospective Randomized Milrinone Survival Evaluation (PROMISE) trial, 24-hour ambulatory electrocardiogram recordings were obtained in 1080 patients with Class III or IV heart failure symptoms and left ventricular ejection fraction ≤0.35.[62] Nonsustained VT was present in 61% of patients. The CHF-STAT trial enrolled patients who had >10 PVCs per hour and a left ventricular ejection fraction of ≤0.4.[154] Nonsustained VT was present in 79% of 24-hour recordings obtained in 666 patients. Repeated recordings revealed that nonsustained VT was present at some time in all but 33 of the 666 patients evaluated. Nonsustained VT runs are typically short; only 30% of patients have runs >5 beats in duration.[62] Fast, long runs of nonsustained VT and polymorphic VT should prompt a careful search for possible myocardial ischemia and possible causes of torsades de pointes (see Chapters 1 and 5). Frequent ventricular ectopy and nonsustained VT are markers for increased mortality and sudden death, but appear to reflect the severity of underlying heart failure and ventricular dysfunction, rather than a specific arrhythmia risk.[62,154,155] In the GESICA trial, nonsustained VT predicted total mortality and sudden death independent of functional class.[155] In the PROMISE and CHF-STAT trials, nonsustained VT was associated with a 1.5- to 1.7-fold increase in mortality and approximately twice the risk of sudden death as compared to patients without nonsustained

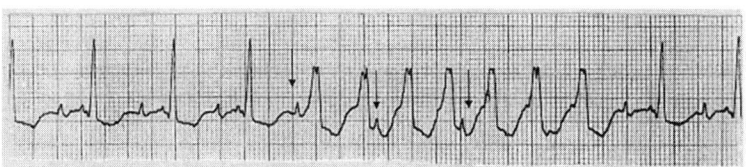

Figure 6–1. An episode of nonsustained VT with AV dissociation (arrows) is shown.

VT. When outcomes were adjusted for the severity of ventricular dysfunction and heart failure, ventricular arrhythmias did not have prognostic significance.[62,154] Furthermore, suppression of nonsustained VT by amiodarone therapy in CHF-STAT did not improve survival. Thus, it appears that ventricular ectopy is a marker of risk, at least in part because it is a marker of the severity of heart failure.

Occasionally ventricular ectopic activity is due to an aggravating factor that requires treatment, or is a marker for hemodynamic deterioration. Hyperkalemia, hypokalemia, hypoxemia, apneic periods during sleep, and myocardial ischemia are potential causes that deserve evaluation when a marked change in the frequency of ectopic activity occurs.[156–159]

Nonsustained Ventricular Tachycardia in Patients with Prior Myocardial Infarction

Amiodarone therapy can be considered for patients with symptomatic ventricular ectopy. A meta-analysis of postinfarction and heart failure trials suggests a small reduction in absolute mortality of 13% and a somewhat greater reduction in sudden death of 23%.[80] However, in patients with prior myocardial infarction, left ventricular ejection fraction <0.40, and nonsustained VT, assessment for implantation of an ICD should be considered. Patients who have reasonably preserved functional capacity, functional Class III or better, are candidates for electrophysiologic testing and ICD implantation if inducible VT is found.

The Multicenter Unsustained Tachycardia Trial (MUSTT) enrolled 2202 patients with prior myocardial infarction, left ventricular ejection fraction <0.4, and nonsustained VT (Table 6–2).[160] Sustained VT was induced at electrophysiology testing in 35% of patients; 704 of these patients were randomized either to a control group that did not receive antiarrhythmic therapy or to a treatment group that received antiarrhythmic drug therapy or an ICD. If electrophysiologic testing failed to induce VT, the patient was followed in a registry. Symptomatic heart failure was not required for trial entry; however, the mean left ventricular ejection fraction was 0.30, Class II or III symptoms were present in 63% of patients, and

Table 6-2

Randomized Trials of ICDs Versus Antiarrhythmic Drugs for Primary Prevention of Sudden Death

	MADIT	CABG Patch	MUSTT
Target population	Post MI	Postcoronary artery bypass grafting	Post MI
Treatment	ICD vs. best available drug therapy	ICD vs. control	ICD vs. EPS-guided drug therapy or no therapy
Patients enrolled	196	900	704
Arrhythmia qualifier	Spontaneous NSVT + inducible, nonsuppressible VT/VF	None (abnormal signal-averaged ECG)	Spontaneous NSVT + inducible VT/VF
LVEF (%) qualifier	≤ 35	<36	≤ 40
CHF qualifier	None	None	None
NYHA II–III (%)	~65	70–75	70–75
NYHA IV (%)	Excluded	Excluded	Excluded
Revascularization (%)	~75	100	56
Mean LVEF (%)	26	27	30
ACE inhibitors (%)	~50	~50	~75
Beta-blockers (%)	~29% ICD vs. 16% drug group	24% ICD vs. 17% control	51% ICD vs. 29% non-ICD
Outcome	*Survival advantage in ICD group*	*No difference in survival*	*Survival advantage in ICD group*
Total mortality rate	16% ICD vs. 34% drug @ 1 year (hazard ratio 0.46)	27% ICD vs. 24% control @ 4 years	24% ICD vs. 48% no treatment vs. 55% drug treatment @ 5 years
Sudden death rate	3% ICD vs. 13% non-ICD	Not reported	9% ICD vs. 37% non-ICD @ 5 years
Comments	Drug therapy: 80% amiodarone, 11% Class IA, 9% no antiarrhythmic drug at discharge	Amiodarone 4% in both groups; Class IA drugs 17% ICD vs. 12% control	Most patients randomized to drug therapy were taking Class IA agents

VF = ventricular fibrillation; NSVT = nonsustained ventricular tachycardia; VT = ventricular tachycardia; LVEF = left ventricular ejection fraction; CHF = congestive heart failure; NYHA = New York Heart Association Functional Class; RR = risk reduction; EPS = electrophysiology study; MI = myocardial infarction.

50 CLINICAL APPROACHES TO TACHYARRHYTHMIAS

72% to 75% were treated with ACE inhibitors. Beta-blockers were administered to 51% of patients in the no antiarrhythmic therapy group and to 29% in the arrhythmia therapy group. The 5-year rate of sudden death or resuscitation from cardiac arrest was 32% for the patients who did not receive antiarrhythmic therapy compared to 25% for those assigned to antiarrhythmic therapy (relative risk, 0.73; 95% confidence interval, 0.53 to 0.99). The benefit of treatment was due to ICDs, which were implanted in 46% of patients in the treatment group. Patients with an ICD had a 5-year rate of sudden death or cardiac arrest of 9% compared to 37% for patients treated with antiarrhythmic drugs. Although ICD therapy was not directly compared to treatment with amiodarone, it seems likely that ICDs provide better protection against sudden death, as has been observed in the secondary prevention trials of cardiac arrest survivors (Chapter 4).[76,93–95] A smaller primary prevention trial (MADIT) enrolled 196 patients with prior infarction, left ventricular ejection fraction ≤0.35, and inducible VT at EPS that was not suppressed by administration of intravenous procainamide.[161] Patients were randomized to ICD versus antiarrhythmic drug therapy (amiodarone in 74% of the drug treatment group). Survival was better in the ICD group (hazard ratio 0.46, 95% confidence interval, 0.26 to 0.82).

Whether recent surgical revascularization should influence selection of patients for an ICD is not clear. The Coronary Artery Bypass Graft (CABG) Patch Trial enrolled patients undergoing coronary artery bypass surgery who had a left ventricular ejection fraction <36% and an abnormal signal-averaged electrocardiogram (Table 6–2).[162] Patients were randomized to receive an ICD (an epicardial lead system) at the time or surgery or to no ICD. During follow-up, there was no difference in mortality even though ICD shocks were frequent. One possible explanation is that coronary artery revascularization reduces sudden death risk.

Based on available evidence, patients with heart failure due to coronary artery disease, in whom the severity of heart failure and other co-morbidities do not preclude an ICD (see Chapter 3), should undergo electrophysiologic testing if they have nonsustained VT and left ventricular ejection fraction <0.4. ICDs are recommended for those who have inducible VT.

Whether patients with depressed ventricular function who do not have inducible VT benefit from an ICD is not known. In the

MUSTT registry, patients who have depressed ventricular function and nonsustained VT but who do not have inducible VT have a lower but still important sudden death risk of approximately 6% per year for the first 2 years compared to a risk of 9% per year for those with inducible VT.[163] Whether an ICD would reduce sudden death in these patients is the subject of ongoing trials. The preliminary report of the MADIT II trial suggests that all patients (excluding those with Class IV symptoms) who have coronary artery disease and a left ventricular ejection fraction <0.3 may benefit.

Nonsustained Ventricular Tachycardia in Patients with Nonischemic Cardiomyopathy

In unselected patients with nonischemic causes of heart failure and nonsustained VT who have not had an episode of sustained VT or syncope, electrophysiologic testing with programmed ventricular stimulation is not useful for risk stratification. Programmed stimulation induced sustained monomorphic VT in only 7% of 274 such patients reported in 7 series.[20,21,164–168] During average follow-up periods of less than 2 years, 12% of patients died suddenly. The results of programmed stimulation were not predictive of outcome.

Electrophysiologic study with programmed stimulation should be considered for some patients with nonischemic dilated cardiomyopathy, such as those who have symptoms suggesting an arrhythmia that has not been documented with electrocardiographic recording. Supraventricular or ventricular arrhythmias may be inducible and confirmed as the cause. Occasionally an EPS is helpful in suggesting a diagnosis when a cardiomyopathic process associated with scar-related arrhythmias such as arrhythmogenic right ventricular cardiomyopathy, cardiac involvement with sarcoidosis, or Chagas' disease is suspected.[23–30] In these disorders, ventricular mapping often identifies areas of low amplitude and abnormal electrograms, indicating regions of scar, and VT may be inducible.

Whether therapy targeting arrhythmias is warranted in this population is controversial and the subject of ongoing study. In the GESICA trial, patients with heart failure were randomized to receive amiodarone or no antiarrhythmic drug therapy.[77,90,155] Amiodarone reduced mortality from 41% to 33.5% and sudden death from 15% to 12% (relative risk reduction, 27%). Only 39% of patients had a history of prior myocardial infarction in this trial, and most had nonischemic causes of heart failure. In contrast, in the CHF-STAT trial, in which approximately 71% of patients had coronary artery disease, no difference was found in mortality rates between amiodarone-treated and placebo groups.[78]

The AMIOVERT trial randomized patients with nonischemic dilated cardiomyopathy, nonsustained VT, and left ventricular ejection fraction <0.35 to therapy with amiodarone or an ICD.[169] The preliminary report of this trial found no difference in survival between the two groups.

Thus, whether ICDs will improve survival in patients with nonischemic cardiomyopathy who have not had syncope or a prior cardiac arrest has not yet been proven. Amiodarone may have benefit in some patients. In the GESICA trial, benefit of amiodarone was confined to those patients who had a relatively rapid resting heart rate (>90 beats/min) after optimization of heart failure therapies, suggesting that slowing of heart rate may have conferred benefit.[77,81] These trials were conducted, however, before therapy with beta-blockers became routine. Whether the addition of amiodarone to beta-blockers is beneficial, as appears to be the case in patients with prior myocardial infarction, is not known.[80,170]

For the present, we recommend chronic therapy with amiodarone to patients with symptomatic palpitations from nonsustained VT and to patients with nonischemic cardiomyopathy who have relatively rapid resting heart rates, particularly if they are not able to tolerate beta-adrenergic blocking agents. We also consider administration of amiodarone for patients who have a very high density of ventricular ectopy, such as incessant ventricular bigeminy, based on the unproven assumption that suppression of ectopic activity may improve hemodynamic performance in some of these patients.[171]

Heart Rate Variability

Beat-to-beat variability of individual R-R intervals reflects activity and function of the autonomic nervous system, sinus node, and circulating humoral factors.[35,172] Analysis of heart rate variability is affected by a number of technical factors, including the duration of the electrocardiogram recording, ventricular and atrial ectopy and the methods used for excluding these beats, and the subject's activity during the recording. These and other factors can cause misleading or unreliable results.[35,173]

Several methods of analysis are available. Frequency domain measures calculate the power spectral density and typically identify three main components: a very low-frequency component below 0.04 Hz, a low-frequency component from 0.04 to 0.15 Hz, and a high-frequency component between 0.15 and 0.4 Hz. The high-frequency component matches the frequency of respiration and respiratory sinus arrhythmia and largely reflects parasympathetic activity.[174] The low-frequency component appears to reflect both sympathetic and parasympathetic influences. Time domain analyses calculate one or more measures of the variance of R-R intervals, such as the standard deviation of all R-R intervals. Nonlinear analyses have also been used.[31]

Diminished beat-to-beat heart rate variability is a marker of sympathetic activation and increased circulating norepinephrine that occurs in heart failure.[31–34] It parallels severity of heart failure, ventricular dysfunction, ambient ventricular ectopy, and total mortality, and in some but not all studies, sudden death.[10,11,31,36,175–181] In a study of 433 out-patients with chronic functional Class I, II, or III heart failure (mean left ventricular ejection fraction 0.41 ± 0.14), a time domain measure of heart rate variability was a predictor of total mortality and death from progressive heart failure, but did not predict sudden death.[11]

Thus, in chronic heart failure, depressed heart rate variability is a marker of impaired ventricular function and more severe heart failure. It is not sufficiently specific for predicting sudden death to be useful for selecting patients for ICD implantation or other arrhythmia therapies.

AV Block

In a study of 94 patients with nonischemic dilated cardiomyopathy, first-degree AV block or any AV block on 24-hour Holter recordings was associated with a 4.6-fold increase in sudden

54 CLINICAL APPROACHES TO TACHYARRHYTHMIAS

death risk.[53] Whether the deaths were due to bradyarrhythmias or ventricular arrhythmias is not clear. Permanent pacing should be considered for appropriate indications.[182]

ST-T and QT Interval Analyses

Downregulation of repolarizing potassium currents in ventricular hypertrophy and heart failure prolongs action potential duration, the QT interval, and potentially increases susceptibility to torsades de pointes (Chapter 1). Several methods of analysis of the ST-T wave segment and QT interval of the surface electrocardiogram are being evaluated as potential markers of arrhythmia risk in heart failure.

QT Interval Dispersion

Differences in recovery times across the ventricle promote reentrant arrhythmias. QT interval dispersion is the difference between the longest and shortest QT interval measured from different leads of the body surface electrocardiogram. QT dispersion has been proposed as a measure of dispersion of ventricular recovery times.[183-186] Although initial studies were promising, subsequent evaluations have shown that the measurement is unreliable. QT dispersion was not related to mortality or arrhythmic death in 703 heart failure patients entered into the Danish Investigations of Arrhythmia and Mortality on Dofetilide-CHF (Diamond-CHF) study.[184]

Beat-to-Beat QT Interval Variability

Berger and coworkers developed a sophisticated algorithm for quantifying beat-to-beat variability in the QT interval.[186] Beat-to-beat variation (normalized for heart rate) was increased in patients with dilated cardiomyopathy from ischemic or nonischemic causes compared to healthy controls and was associated with more severe symptoms among the heart failure patients.[186]

In patients referred for electrophysiologic evaluation, QT interval variability was associated with a history of sustained ventricular arrhythmias.[187] The utility of this measure for selecting high-risk heart failure patients for therapy has not yet been determined.

T-Wave Alternans

Beat-to-beat alternation in T-wave amplitude is a harbinger of VF during myocardial ischemia, in the long QT syndrome, and during rapid pacing.[188–190] Alternans may reflect heterogeneity of recovery and conduction. Low-amplitude (microvolt) beat-to-beat oscillations in T-wave amplitude when heart rate is increased by pacing or exercise can be quantitated with a commercially available system. Abnormal T-wave alternans has been associated with inducible ventricular arrhythmias at EPS and with recurrent spontaneous arrhythmias.[191–197] It also appears to be a marker for worse heart failure and ventricular function. In 221 patients with dilated cardiomyopathy, patients with abnormal T-wave alternans had more severely depressed left ventricular function and dilation compared to those without abnormal T-wave alternans.[198] To achieve adequate sensitivity, it appears that heart rate must be increased to >100 beats/min, which may be difficult to achieve in some heart failure patients.[191,195] The utility of this measure for selecting high-risk heart failure patients for therapy has not yet been determined.

Summary

Ongoing primary prevention trials will provide further guidance for management of patients with heart failure who have not had a cardiac arrest, sustained VT, or syncope. Current evidence supports ICD implantation for high-risk patients with coronary artery disease who have the additional risk factors discussed above. Adequate selection of the highest risk patients who would benefit from an arrhythmia treatment strategy has not yet been achieved for other patient groups.

7

Syncope

Syncope is the sudden and transient loss of consciousness accompanied by the loss of postural tone.[199–201] Systolic blood pressure less than 70 mm Hg or interruption of cerebral blood flow for 8–10 seconds usually results in syncope.[202] Because cerebral blood flow decreases with aging, the elderly are more prone to syncope.[202] The occurrence of syncope is a marker of high risk for sudden death in patients with advanced heart failure.[203–206]

There are a variety of causes of syncope and diagnosis is often challenging (Table 7–1). Among 491 consecutive patients with advanced heart failure, Middlekauff and coworkers found that 12% had a history of syncope.[206] In 45% of patients, syncope was attributed to a cardiac arrhythmia, and no clear cause was identified in 30% of patients. In 25% of patients, syncope was attributed to orthostatic hypotension and other noncardiac causes. The rate of sudden death during the following year was 45%. The sudden death risk was similar for patients with identifiable cardiac causes and presumptively identified noncardiac causes of syncope, suggesting that even when an apparently benign explanation is found, patients with heart failure and syncope remain at high risk for sudden death.

The initial evaluation of a patient with heart failure and syncope is critically important. It should include a careful history of the event with a search for situational or provocative factors. Occurrence with a sudden change in posture suggests orthostatic hypotension, which may be aggravated by vasodilating drugs, beta-blockers, and diuresis. Orthostatic hypotension, however, is often present in patients who are ultimately diagnosed with other etiologies of syncope and should not preclude further appropriate diagnostic testing.[207] Incontinence, injury, and clonic-tonic muscle activity are nonspecific features of syncope that do not help distinguish syncope from a seizure.[208,209]

Table 7-1
Differential Diagnosis of Syncope[199–201]

Cardiovascular
Arrhythmia
  Bradyarrhythmia
    sinus node disease
    AV node disease
    drug-induced
    pacemaker malfunction

  Tachyarrhythmia
    ventricular arrhythmias
    supraventricular arrhythmias

Low Cardiac Output
  obstruction to flow
    aortic stenosis
    mitral stenosis
    tricuspid stenosis
    hypertrophic cardiomyopathy
    atrial myxoma
    pulmonary stenosis
    pulmonary embolism
    pulmonary hypertension
  cardiac tamponade
  aortic dissection
  pump failure (cardiomyopathy, MI)

Disorders of Autonomic Control
Autonomic Insufficiency
  Diabetes mellitus
  Parkinson's disease
  Amyloidosis
  Primary
Reflex-Mediated
  Neurocardiogenic (vasovagal/vasodepressor)
  Carotid sinus hypersensitivity
  Situational (cough, defecation, micturition, swallow)
  Neuralgia (trigeminal, glossopharyngeal)

Neurological
  cerebrovascular disease
    (CVA, TIA)
  seizure
  hyperventilation
  migraine
  narcolepsy
  subclavian steal
Orthostatic Hypotension
  volume depletion
  medication related

Psychiatric
  anxiety disorder/panic disorder
  major depression
    somatization
    Munchausen syndrome
  substance abuse

Metabolic
  hypoadrenalism
  hypoglycemia
  hypothyroidism
  hypoxia

AV = atrioventricular; CVA = cerebrovascular accident; MI = myocardial infarction; TIA = transient ischemic attack.

Like the history, physical examination should focus on identifying potential clues to the etiology of the syncopal episode. In addition to orthostatic hypotension, other specific signs of cardiovascular disease such as murmurs, bruits, or a blood pressure differential in the arms may suggest valvular disease, hypertrophic cardiomyopathy, vascular disease, or aortic dissection, and should prompt appropriate testing. Diploplia, headache, or other focal signs suggest a neurological abnormality.

While almost half of the patients presenting with syncope have significant electrocardiographic abnormalities at baseline including left ventricular hypertrophy, evidence of prior myocardial infarction, or bifascicular block, the initial electrocardiogram establishes a cause of syncope, such as AV block, in fewer than 10% of cases.[199–201,210] Careful assessment of the 12-lead ECG for QT prolongation is warranted and may suggest the possibility of torsades de pointes. The prevalence of acute myocardial infarction or ischemia in patients presenting with syncope and without chest pain is ~7%, and the vast majority of these patients have an abnormal ECG.[211] Although unlikely to reveal the precise cause of syncope, the ECG is an important part of the diagnostic evaluation and helps guide further management.

Long-term electrocardiogram monitoring can be performed to diagnose ventricular arrhythmias, supraventricular arrhythmias, or bradyarrhythmias, but it generally has a low yield. The majority of patients (~65%) have no arrhythmia and no symptoms even during prolonged Holter monitoring and this testing can result in a delay of definitive therapy.[212] Implantable monitors can be used in patients with rare but recurrent unexplained syncope. These devices automatically record rhythm abnormalities and can be patient-activated. In heart failure patients, these devices may best be reserved for patients who do not receive a pacemaker or ICD after a negative diagnostic evaluation (including EPS).[213]

When the cause of syncope is uncertain after the history, physical examination, and electrocardiogram, EPS should be considered. This test is well established for detecting ventricular arrhythmias and supraventricular arrhythmias but is less sensitive for detecting bradyarrhythmias.[213–215] "Positive" findings considered an indication of the cause of syncope include:[214–216]

1. Inducible sustained monomorphic VT
2. Inducible sustained supraventricular tachycardia causing hypotension
3. Prolonged corrected sinus node recovery time (>1000 ms)
4. Markedly prolonged HV interval >100 ms
5. Infranodal block either spontaneously or with atrial pacing.

Inducible nonsustained VT, sustained polymorphic VT/VF, or an HV interval that is only moderately prolonged (75–100 ms) are nonspecific findings that require clinical judgment for interpretation.

Patients with syncope and inducible VT at EPS have mortality rates similar to patients with documented sustained ventricular tachyarrhythmias and a similarly high incidence of subsequent spontaneous VT.[205,217,218]

It is important to note that a negative EPS does not always exclude the possibility of a serious arrhythmia. In particular, patients with nonischemic causes of cardiomyopathy and unexplained syncope often have false negative electrophysiologic studies. Knight and coworkers implanted ICDs in 14 patients with nonischemic cardiomyopathy, unexplained syncope, and a negative EPS.[205] During an average follow-up of 2 years, half of the patients received therapy from the ICD for VT or VF. Of 639 consecutive patients with nonischemic cardiomyopathy referred for heart transplantation reported by Fonarow and coworkers, 147 (23%) had a history of syncope.[203] Twenty-five of these patients received an ICD; 40% received an appropriate shock for VT and none died suddenly during a mean follow-up of 22 months. Of the 122 patients who had a history of syncope but did not receive an ICD, 15% died suddenly during follow-up. Actuarial survival at 2 years was 84.9% with ICD therapy and 66.9% with conventional therapy.

Patients with ischemic cardiomyopathy and negative electrophysiologic studies also remain at risk for sudden death, probably due to false negative EPS results.[163,219] Implantation of an ICD is recommended for most patients with heart failure and unexplained syncope.[203–205]

Summary

Syncope is a common and challenging problem in patients with heart failure. In most patients, it indicates a high risk of sudden death from arrhythmias. While a thorough evaluation is warranted, the sensitivity of diagnostic testing for predicting sudden death is limited. In the absence of a clear, benign, or treated cause of syncope, ICD therapy should be strongly considered.

8
Bradyarrhythmias and Pacing

Bradyarrhythmias due to conduction system disease cause syncope and some sudden deaths in patients with heart failure.[39,53] Conduction disturbances (AV block, and prolonged QRS duration) are common in patients with heart failure, generally reflect the severity of the underlying heart disease, and are markers of increased mortality.[51–53] In a series of 94 patients with nonischemic dilated cardiomyopathy, first- or second-degree AV block was observed on ambulatory electrocardiograms in 28% of patients and was associated with a greater than 4-fold increase in risk of sudden death.[53] Bradycardia can also aggravate heart failure.

Bradyarrhythmias occasionally have a secondary cause, including hyperkalemia, hypoxemia, sleep apnea, myocardial ischemia, or are a reflex response to pain or discomfort (Table 8–1).[156–159] Therapy with beta-adrenergic blocking agents or amiodarone are also common aggravating factors. Pacing support for bradyarrhythmias is indicated for symptomatic bradycardias when a secondary factor cannot be corrected. Whether the benefit of beta-adrenergic blockers or therapy with amiodarone is sufficient to justify implantation of a pacemaker to allow continued administration of the drug is a decision that must be made on an individual basis. For patients treated chronically with amiodarone, withdrawal of the drug is often not feasible due to the very long time required for the drug to be excreted and for the effects to dissipate once the patient has accumulated tissue stores of the drug.

Dedicated Bradycardia Pacing System Versus an Implantable Defibrillator

ICDs that incorporate essentially all of the features of dedicated bradycardia pacemakers are now available. Because pa-

Table 8–1

Causes and Aggravating Factors for Bradyarrhythmias

Primary bradyarrhythmias
  sick sinus syndrome
  atrioventricular block
Reflex or neurally mediated
  neurocardiogenic
  response to an acute illness:
    myocardial ischemia
    stroke
    aortic dissection
    exsanguination
    respiratory arrest/apnea (including sleep apnea)
    cardiac tamponade
Drugs
  digoxin
  calcium channel blockers (particularly verapamil and diltiazem)
  all antiarrhythmic drugs (particularly amiodarone, sotalol, propafenone, flecainide)
  beta-blockers
  centrally acting sympatholytic agents: (e.g., clonidine, alphamethyldopa)
Acute myocardial ischemia
Hyperkalemia
Hypoglycemia

tients with heart failure are also at risk for sudden death from ventricular arrhythmias, patients who require bradycardia pacing are often candidates for an ICD that will also treat VT or fibrillation. The perceived arrhythmia risk and general prognosis from the standpoint of heart failure severity are important considerations in this decision (see Chapter 3; Figure 8–1). If both bradycardia pacing and protection from VT or fibrillation are required, implantation of a single ICD rather than both an ICD and dedicated bradycardia pacing systems is preferable to minimize the implanted hardware and to avoid potential adverse interactions between the pacemaker and the ICD that may cause spurious arrhythmia detection or prevent appropriate detection of an arrhythmia.

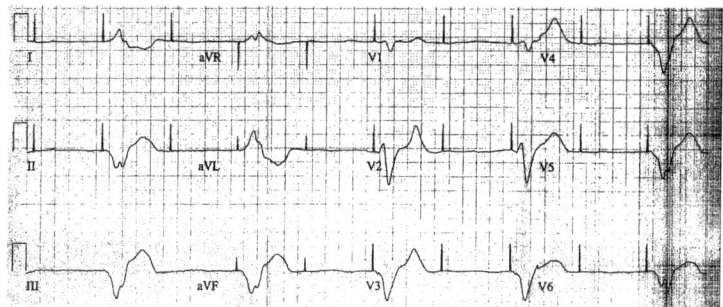

Figure 8–1. Loss of ventricular pacing capture due to hyperkalemia in a patient with heart failure and a permanent pacemaker.

There are some potentially significant differences between dedicated bradycardia pacing systems and ICDs that are relevant in individual patients. Bradycardia pulse generators are much smaller than an ICD and have longer battery life, typically exceeding 10 years, compared to 6–8 years projected for many ICDs. As discussed below, AV pacing with an ICD generally mandates ventricular capture, without the possibility of allowing intrinsic AV conduction, in contrast to some dedicated bradycardia pacing systems.

Dual Chamber Atrioventricular Pacing Versus Single Chamber Ventricular Pacing

When sinus rhythm is present, AV synchrony can be preserved with dual chamber pacing, requiring placement of an atrial lead as well as the ventricular lead.[104] Maintenance of AV synchrony is theoretically desirable from a hemodynamic standpoint, although not much data exist to support this common clinical perception.[220] Maintenance of AV synchrony by atrial or AV pacing was compared to single chamber pacing in 1474 patients (not specifically a heart failure population) in the Canadian Trial of Physiologic Pacing (CTOPP). Preservation of AV synchrony reduced the incidence of atrial fibrillation by 18% compared to single chamber ventricular pacing, but did not reduce mortality or the incidence of stroke.[221] Prevention of atrial fibrillation may, however, be particularly relevant to patients with heart failure. Although data in heart failure populations are limited, we advocate dual chamber pacing rather than single chamber VVI pacing in heart failure.

The optimal AV delay for pacing in heart failure is controversial. Short AV delays (<120 ms) may occasionally improve hemodynamics by reducing presystolic mitral regurgitation, but the hemodynamic improvement is inconsistent and pacing to regulate the AV delay is not in itself an indication for pacing.[222,223]

The consequences of pacing to maintain AV synchrony are complicated by the potential impact of right ventricular pacing on ventricular function. "Physiologic" DDD pacing with a dual chamber pacemaker is not equivalent to "physiologic" pacing achieved with atrial pacing with intact AV conduction (AAI pacing). Both maintain AV synchrony. With DDD pacing, ventricular activation begins from the ventricular pacing site, most commonly at the right ventricular apex. In contrast, with atrial pacing with AV conduction, ventricular activation occurs from the His-Purkinje system. Evidence is increasing that slow interventricular conduction, indicated by the presence of a prolonged QRS duration and which can be produced by right ventricular pacing, can have an adverse effect on ventricular performance and may worsen heart failure in some circumstances.[105–107,222,224–228] Right ventricular pacing can reduce left ventricular ejection fraction, increase mitral regurgitation, reduce regional myocardial perfusion of the left ventricular septum, and cause thinning and myofibrillar cellular disarray in portions of the ventricle that are activated early. When the QRS complex is wide, with left bundle branch block, during AV conduction, right ventricular pacing may be less of a concern, since the activation sequence may be similar. However, if the native QRS is narrow, right ventricular apical pacing may have an adverse effect in some patients. An adverse effect of right ventricular pacing has been suggested to explain the association of permanent pacing with death from pump failure observed in a retrospective analysis of patients with advanced heart failure, and with total mortality in the AVID trial registry.[229–231] Alternatively, the need for a pacemaker may simply be a marker of more advanced heart disease.

Although these concerns are not yet resolved, we prefer to avoid right ventricular apical pacing when there is normal ventricular activation (i.e., narrow QRS duration). Optimal pacing and sensing operation in current dual chamber ICD systems necessitates short AV intervals with DDD pacing, which results in ventricular pacing from the right ventricular apex. In patients with dual chamber ICDs who have intact AV conduction backup, VVI pacing below the intrinsic heart rate, which results in supraventricular conduction and rare ventricular pacing, might be preferable to DDD chronic right ventricular apical pacing.

Ventricular Resynchronization Therapy: Biventricular Pacing

A prolonged time for ventricular activation can have an adverse effect on ventricular performance, similar to that produced by pacing from the right ventricular apex. With markedly prolonged activation, portions of the ventricle begin contracting while regions that are activated later are still relaxed, potentially cushioning some of the initial force of contraction. Left ventricular pacing or simultaneous left ventricular and right ventricular pacing (Figure 8-2) has the potential to achieve a more physiological sequence of ventricular activation. In patients with depressed systolic function and prolonged QRS durations (typically exceeding 150 ms), initial data suggest that pacing from the left ventricle or simultaneously from the left ventricle and right ventricle can improve ventricular performance and functional capacity.[232-240] Sympathetic nervous system activation and ambient ventricular arrhythmias are reduced in some patients.[236,241,242]

Left ventricular pacing can be achieved by placing a pacing lead through the coronary sinus and into the distal ramifications of the epicardial venous system. The hemodynamic effect is dependent not only on the site of left ventricular pacing, but also on the presence of coordinated atrial activity and optimization of the AV interval.

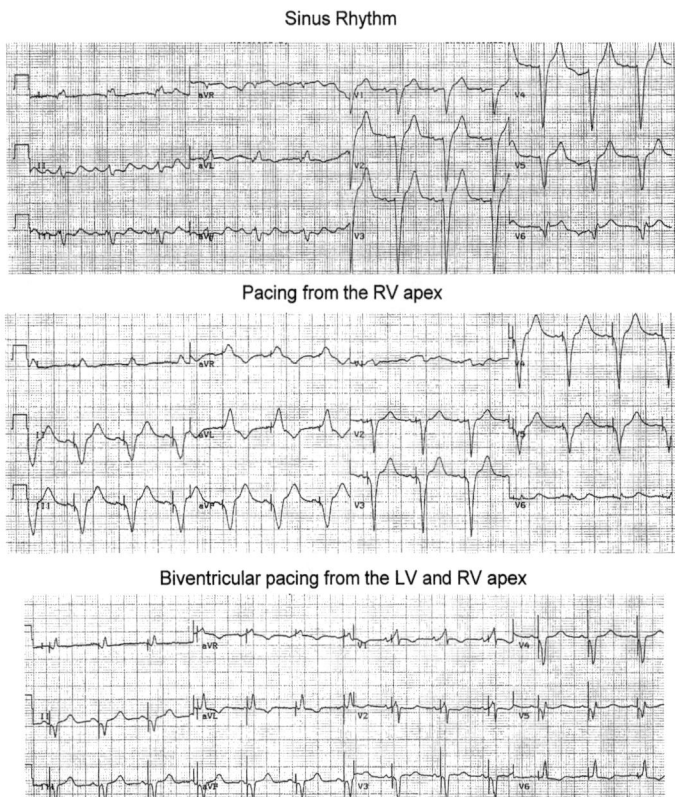

Figure 8–2. The effects of right ventricular pacing (middle panel) and biventricular pacing from simultaneous pacing at the basal lateral left ventricle and right ventricular apex (lower panel) on the 12-lead electrocardiogram in a patient with advanced heart failure is shown. In this patient, the QRS duration is 170 ms during sinus rhythm with left bundle branch block, 210 ms during DDD pacing from the right ventricular apex, and 150 ms during biventricular pacing. The sinus rhythm electrocardiogram showing left bundle branch block is at the top.

Multicenter Insync Randomized Clinical Evaluation

The Multicenter Insync Randomized Clinical Evaluation (MIRACLE) trial evaluated biventricular pacing in patients with chronic dilated heart failure, left ventricular ejection fraction ≤0.35, left ventricular end-diastolic dimension >55 mm, functional Class III or IV symptoms, and a QRS duration >130 ms.[243] Stable medical therapy for heart failure for at least 1 month was required, excluding patients with recent decompensation. Patients with atrial arrhythmias were also excluded. Implantation of a three-lead biventricular pacing system (epicardial left ventricle via the coronary venous system, right ventricle, and right atrium) was attempted. Implantation was successful in 266 patients (93% of patients attempted) who had an average age of 64 ± 11 years, average left ventricular ejection fraction of 0.22 ± 0.06, and average left ventricular end-diastolic dimension of 69.5 ± 9 mm. The majority of patients (91%) had functional Class III symptoms at study entry. The mean QRS duration was 165 ± 19 ms. Patients were randomized to cardiac resynchronization therapy (CRT) with biventricular pacing or to the control group whose device was programmed for backup bradycardia pacing from the right ventricular pacing site alone (VVI mode) at a slow rate (30 beats/min), such that there would be little or no ventricular pacing. After 6 months, patients in the control group crossed over to biventricular pacing. The patients and treating staff, with the exception of the implanting electrophysiologist, were blinded to the mode of pacing. Treatment with angiotensin-converting enzyme inhibitors or angiotensin receptor-blocking drugs was similar in both groups (87% and 94%, respectively). Beta-blockers were administered more frequently to the CRT patients (60% compared to 48% for the control group), although the difference was not statistically significant. Mortality was not an endpoint of the trial. During 6 months of follow-up, 10 patients died in the control group and 8 died in the CRT group. Another 4 patients failed to complete the 6-month follow-up period. Preliminary data were reported for the 119 patients in the control group and 125 in the treatment group who completed 6 months of follow-up.

CRT improved functional capacity (the primary outcome). After 1 month of follow-up, the 6-minute walk distance increased by an average of 39 meters from the baseline evaluation and remained improved at the 3- and 6-month assessments. In contrast, the 6-minute walk distance did not change appreciably over the 6 months in the control group. The improvement in functional capacity was further supported by analysis of the secondary endpoints in 80 control and 87 treatment group patients. Maximal oxygen capacity (peak VO_2) improved from baseline in the CRT group, but not in the control group. Total exercise duration improved in both groups but to a greater extent in the CRT group, in whom exercise duration increased by more than 100 seconds compared to their baseline ($P<0.001$). Quality of life (assessed from the Minnesota Living with Heart Failure Questionnaire) improved in both groups, but the magnitude of improvement was greater in the CRT group ($P=0.013$). Echocardiograms in a cohort of 124 patients showed an improvement in LVEF by 6% from baseline ($P<0.001$) and a reduction in LVED dimension by 5 mm from baseline ($P<0.001$) for CRT patients and no change in the control group.

Although it is a preliminary report and it appears that the CRT group may be less ill than those randomized to the control group as indicated by the better initial 6-minute walk distance at baseline and more beta-blocker use, some of these concerns will likely be addressed in the planned future analysis of the control group patients after they are crossed over to CRT in the unblinded phase of the study.

The initial results of the MIRACLE trial suggest that biventricular pacing improves symptoms and exercise capacity in patients with functional Class III and IV heart failure who have sinus rhythm and QRS duration >130 ms. The benefit appears to be maintained during 6 months of follow-up. Further study is needed to confirm benefit, to determine the durability of the effect long term, and to clarify which patients are most likely to benefit. The impact on mortality is not yet known. Devices that combine biventricular pacing to treat heart failure with ICD capability to treat ventricular arrhythmias hold promise for improving functional capacity and survival.

Summary

Permanent pacing is often needed in patients with heart failure due to bradyarrhythmias that are symptomatic or that limit administration of other therapies felt to be necessary, such as beta-adrenergic blockers or amiodarone. Whether implantation of a pacemaker to allow administration of a beta-block for patients without symptoms requiring this medication is better than withholding the medication and avoiding a pacemaker is not known. AV sequential pacing is preferred when sinus rhythm is present. For many patients with heart failure, implantation of an ICD that incorporates the desired bradycardia pacing functions is a reasonable consideration. Cardiac resynchronization therapy with biventricular pacing can be considered for patients with advanced heart failure and prolonged QRS duration. Technical improvements with these systems can be anticipated and further trials will help define those patients most likely to benefit.

9

Atrial Fibrillation and Flutter

Atrial Fibrillation

The prevalence of atrial fibrillation increases with the severity of heart failure (Figure 9–1). Atrial fibrillation is found in 6% of patients with mild heart failure and in more than 40% of patients with advanced heart failure (Figure 9–1).[15,57,75,244–248] The potential adverse effects of atrial fibrillation include loss of AV synchrony, rapid or slow ventricular rate responses that are no longer under optimal physiological control, variability in time for cardiac filling due to oscillations of R-R intervals, and risk of thromboembolism.[71,75,249–251] In some but not all studies, patients with atrial fibrillation have increased mortality rates and more frequent hospitalizations compared to those heart failure patients who do not have atrial fibrillation.[75,244,245,248,252] Atrial fibrillation may be a marker for worse outcome because it is another marker for increased severity of heart failure or it may directly impact on outcome. It is likely that both factors contribute to the observed association with mortality.

Management

Patients with atrial fibrillation and heart failure are at increased risk of stroke; anticoagulation with warfarin is warranted.[42,253,254] There is also uniform agreement that adequate control of heart rate is important. Whether attempting to restore and maintain sinus rhythm is better than simply controlling the ventricular rate and maintaining anticoagulation is not known.[71,255] In the CHF-STAT trial, patients who converted from atrial fibrillation to sinus rhythm during therapy with amiodarone

Arrhythmias in Heart Failure   71

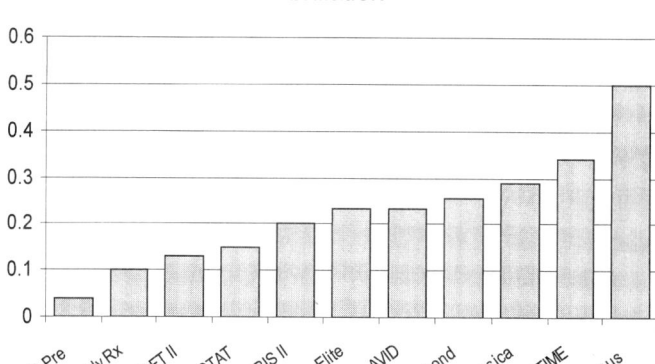

Figure 9–1. The incidence of atrial fibrillation observed in recent heart failure and arrhythmia trials is shown.

had better survival rates compared to those who did not convert.[246] Similarly, patients treated with dofetilide who achieved sinus rhythm had fewer hospitalizations for heart failure exacerbations.[15] Sinus rhythm may be beneficial, or alternatively, patients who remained in atrial fibrillation may have had more severe heart failure.

For patients with a first episode of atrial fibrillation and those with symptomatic paroxysms of atrial fibrillation, antiarrhythmic drug therapy to attempt to maintain sinus rhythm is reasonable. Class I antiarrhythmic drugs (e.g., quinidine, flecainide, propafenone, procainamide, disopyramide, moricizine) should be avoided because their negative inotropic effects and potential proarrhythmic effects may increase mortality (Chapter 2).[74] Amiodarone (which is not specifically approved for this indication), dofetilide, and sotalol are the major antiarrhythmic drug options.[15] Amiodarone is most likely to be effective.[84,92,256] In a randomized trial of patients with atrial fibrillation without heart failure, maintenance of sinus rhythm for 1 year was achieved in 69% of patients treated with amiodarone compared to 39% of those treated with sotalol or the Class I antiarrhythmic drug propafenone.[92] Sotalol blocks the same cardiac potassium channel as dofetilide, but also has beta-adrenergic blocking properties. In the

DIAMOND trial, 12% of patients who had atrial fibrillation on entry to the study converted to sinus rhythm by 1 month when treated with dofetilide; only 1% of atrial fibrillation patients in the placebo group converted to sinus rhythm.[15] Dofetilide also reduced the risk of recurrent atrial fibrillation once sinus rhythm had been restored (hazard ratio, 0.35).[15] Amiodarone and dofetilide have not been directly compared. Amiodarone depresses both sinus and AV node function. Attention to the possibility of bradyarrhythmias is important and warrants discontinuation or adjustment of therapies that slow heart rate in up to a third of patients when amiodarone is initiated.[84]

When sinus rhythm cannot be maintained, adequate rate control during atrial fibrillation is of paramount importance.[79,138,249,254,257,258] A poorly controlled ventricular rate can exacerbate heart failure and contribute to further deterioration in ventricular function. A resting heart rate below 80 to 90 beats/min and remaining below 100/min with comfortable ambulation is a reasonable goal. Beta-adrenergic blockers and digoxin are the first-line options for rate control.[254] Digoxin is less effective when sympathetic tone is elevated, but useful because it lacks adverse hemodynamic effects in heart failure. The calcium channel blockers diltiazem and verapamil effectively depress conduction through the AV node and effectively diminish heart rate, but should be avoided in patients with advanced heart failure because of their negative inotropic effects and potential for increasing mortality in patients with heart failure due to coronary artery disease.[259] Amiodarone is an effective drug for rate control but other agents are preferable because of the associated toxicities of amiodarone.

When adequate rate control cannot be achieved with pharmacological means, catheter ablation of the AV junction with implantation of a permanent pacemaker should be considered. AV junction ablation achieves rate control and regularizes the heart rhythm. The atria continue to fibrillate, necessitating anticoagulation. Although the atrial contribution to ventricular filling is not restored, exertional symptoms and palpitations improve and recurrent hospitalizations may be reduced.[258,260-266] Although symptoms improve, objective demonstrations of improvement in exercise time or oxygen uptake are not usually observed.[249,261] In some patients, left ventricular ejection fraction improves, which may be a consequence of the decrease in rate or a better ability to measure ejection fraction once the heart rate is regularized.[267] Benefits may be due not only to improved control of heart rate, but also to regularization of R to R intervals.[258] New pacing algorithms that attempt to regularize the ventricular rate, "rate smoothing," may make pacing without AV junction ablation an option for some patients in the future.

Two problems are of concern with this procedure. Occasional patients experience a deterioration in heart failure after this procedure.[224,228] A change in ventricular activation sequence produced by right ventricular pacing might be responsible, as discussed above. Patients at greatest risk for hemodynamic deterioration have severely depressed ventricular function and severe mitral regurgitation. Whether biventricular pacing (left ventricular and right ventricular pacing) would reduce this risk is not known. Also, sudden death due to torsades de pointes has occurred after ablation slows the heart rate. Pacing at >90 beats/min for the initial 1 to 3 months after ablation appears to reduce this risk.[268]

Atrial Flutter

Management of atrial flutter is similar to that for atrial fibrillation. Rate control and anticoagulation are important.[254,269–271] Although some studies suggest less risk of left atrial thrombus formation in patients with flutter than that observed in patients with atrial fibrillation, others suggest a similar risk in these two groups.[269–273] Chronic anticoagulation with warfarin is prudent for patients with heart failure and atrial flutter. Recurrent atrial flutter responds poorly to pharmacological therapy, and rate control is often more difficult to achieve than for atrial fibrillation.[274] Persistent rapid rates can contribute to depression of ventricular function and heart failure.[275] Antiarrhythmic drugs that slow the rate of atrial flutter without blocking AV nodal conduction, such as Class I antiarrhythmic drugs, can lead to life-threatening 1:1 AV conduction (Figure 9–2).

The most common form of atrial flutter (Figure 9–2, panel B) is

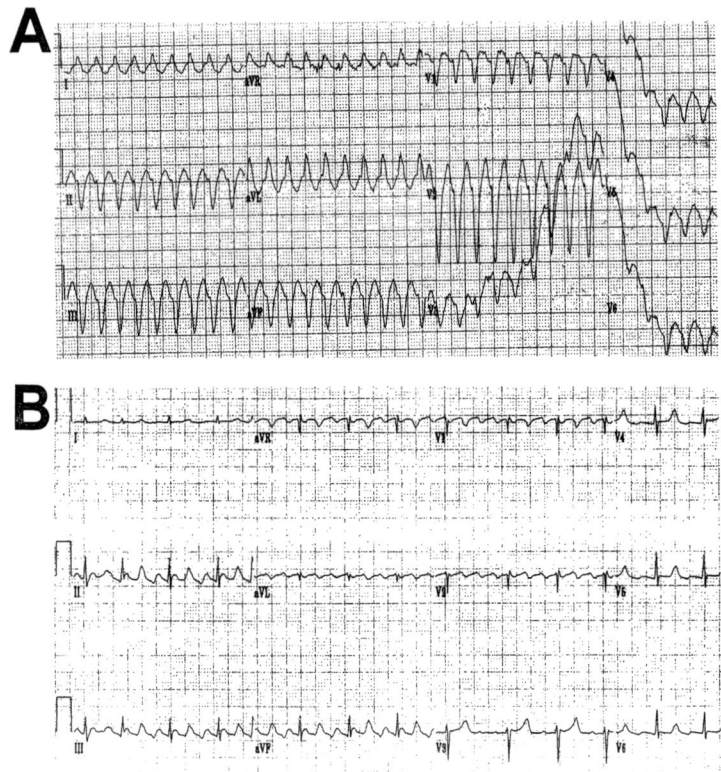

Figure 9–2. In panel A, rapid wide QRS tachycardia due to 1:1 conduction of atrial flutter in a patient who was treated with propafenone. The QRS has a left bundle branch block configuration but a prominent S-wave in V_6 erroneously suggesting VT. Following administration of AV nodal blocking agents (panel B) typical atrial flutter is evident.

due to circulation of a single reentry wavefront around the tricuspid annulus. Radiofrequency catheter ablation is an excellent option for patients with this type of atrial flutter.[276,277] Ablation of the isthmus between the tricuspid valve annulus and the inferior vena cava abolishes atrial flutter in >95% of patients. Procedural risk is minimal. Less commonly, an apparent atrial flutter is due to reentry involving an area of scar in the right or left atrium. Ablation of these types of flutter is more involved, with somewhat lower efficacy. Ablation of flutter in the left atrium is associated with a risk of arterial embolism from left atrial catheter manipulation.

Despite effective ablation of atrial flutter, atrial fibrillation recurs in 20% to 30% of patients within the following 2 years.[277] When atrial flutter develops during chronic drug therapy of atrial fibrillation, ablation of flutter may allow maintenance of sinus rhythm, but drug therapy for prevention of atrial fibrillation is still likely to be required.[278]

Summary

Management of atrial fibrillation and flutter is commonly required in patients with heart failure. Adequate rate control and anticoagulation are warranted for all patients. Attempts to maintain sinus rhythm are reasonable for recent onset and paroxysmal arrhythmias. Amiodarone is the major pharmacological option for fibrillation, and catheter ablation is the major therapeutic option for the common type of atrial flutter. Ongoing trials will provide further guidance as to whether attempts to maintain sinus rhythm will improve outcome.

References

1. Tomaselli GF, Marban E. Electrophysiological remodeling in hypertrophy and heart failure. Cardiovasc Res 1999;42:270–283.
2. Tomaselli GF, Rose J. Molecular aspects of arrhythmias associated with cardiomyopathies. Curr Opin Cardiol 2000;15:202–208.
3. Nabauer M, Kaab S. Potassium channel downregulation in heart failure. Cardiovasc Res 1998;37:324–334.
4. Marban E. Heart failure: the electrophysiologic connection. J Cardiovasc Electrophysiol 1999;10:1425–1428.
5. Jongsma HJ. Modulation of gap junction properties in failing hearts. J Cardiovasc Electrophysiol 1999;10:1421–1424.
6. Priebe L, Beuckelmann DJ. Simulation study of cellular electric properties in heart failure. Circ Res 1998;82:1206–1223.
7. Pogwizd SM, Qi M, Yuan W, et al. Upregulation of Na(+)/Ca(2+) exchanger expression and function in an arrhythmogenic rabbit model of heart failure. Circ Res 1999;85:1009–1019.
8. Middlekauff HR, Stevenson WG, Saxon LA, et al. Amiodarone and torsades de pointes in patients with advanced heart failure. Am J Cardiol 1995;76:499–502.
9. Cooper HA, Dries DL, Davis CE, et al. Diuretics and risk of arrhythmic death in patients with left ventricular dysfunction. Circulation 1999;100:1311–1315.
10. Galinier M, Pathak A, Fourcade J, et al. Depressed low frequency power of heart rate variability as an independent predictor of sudden death in chronic heart failure. Eur Heart J 2000;21:475–482.
11. Nolan J, Batin PD, Andrews R, et al. Prospective study of heart rate variability and mortality in chronic heart failure: results of the United Kingdom Heart Failure Evaluation and Assessment of Risk Trial (UK-HEART). Circulation 1998;98:1510–1516.
12. Pitt B, Zannad F, Remme WJ, et al. The effect of spironolactone on morbidity and mortality in patients with severe heart failure. Randomized Aldactone Evaluation Study Investigators. N Engl J Med 1999;341:709–717.
13. Stevenson WG, Middlekauff HR, Stevenson LW, et al. Significance of aborted cardiac arrest and sustained ventricular

tachycardia in patients referred for treatment therapy of advanced heart failure. Am Heart J 1992;124:123–130.
14. Stevenson WG, Middlekauff HR, Saxon LA. Ventricular arrhythmias in heart failure. In: Zipes DP, Jalife J, eds. Cardiac Electrophysiology: From Cell to Bedside. 2nd ed. Philadelphia: W.B. Saunders Co.; 1995:848–863.
15. Torp-Pedersen C, Moller M, Bloch-Thomsen PE, et al. Dofetilide in patients with congestive heart failure and left ventricular dysfunction. Danish Investigations of Arrhythmia and Mortality on Dofetilide Study Group. N Engl J Med 1999;341:857–865.
16. De Mello WC. Cell coupling and impulse propagation in the failing heart. J Cardiovasc Electrophysiol 1999; 10:1409–1420.
17. de Bakker JM, van Capelle FJ, Janse MJ, et al. Fractionated electrograms in dilated cardiomyopathy: origin and relation to abnormal conduction. J Am Coll Cardiol 1996;27:1071–1078.
18. de Bakker JM, van Capelle FJ, Janse MJ, et al. Slow conduction in the infarcted human heart: "zigzag" course of activation. Circulation 1993;88:915–926.
19. Stevenson WG, Friedman PL, Sager PT, et al. Exploring postinfarction reentrant ventricular tachycardia with entrainment mapping. J Am Coll Cardiol 1997;29:1180–1189.
20. Stevenson WG, Stevenson LW, Weiss J, et al. Inducible ventricular arrhythmias and sudden death during vasodilator therapy of severe heart failure. Am Heart J 1988;116:1447–1454.
21. Turitto G, Ahuja RK, Caref EB, et al. Risk stratification for arrhythmic events in patients with nonischemic dilated cardiomyopathy and nonsustained ventricular tachycardia: role of programmed ventricular stimulation and the signal-averaged electrocardiogram. J Am Coll Cardiol 1994;24:1523–1528.
22. Delacretaz E, Stevenson WG, Ellison KE, et al. Mapping and radiofrequency catheter ablation of the three types of sustained monomorphic ventricular tachycardia in nonischemic heart disease. J Cardiovasc Electrophysiol 2000;11:11–17.
23. Ellison KE, Friedman PL, Ganz LI, et al. Entrainment mapping and radiofrequency catheter ablation of ventricular tachycardia in right ventricular dysplasia. J Am Coll Cardiol 1998;32:724–728.

24. Pinski SL. The right ventricular tachycardias. J Electrocardiol 2000;33:103–114.
25. Corrado D, Basso C, Thiene G, et al. Spectrum of clinicopathologic manifestations of arrhythmogenic right ventricular cardiomyopathy/dysplasia: a multicenter study. J Am Coll Cardiol 1997;30:1512–1520.
26. Case records of the Massachusetts General Hospital. Weekly clinicopathological exercises. Case 20–2000: a 61-year-old man with a wide-complex tachycardia. N Engl J Med 2000;342:1979–1987.
27. Marcus FI, Fontaine G. Arrhythmogenic right ventricular dysplasia/cardiomyopathy: a review. Pacing Clin Electrophysiol 1995;18:1298–1314.
28. Fontaine G, Fontaliran F, Hebert JL, et al. Arrhythmogenic right ventricular dysplasia. Annu Rev Med 1999;50:17–35.
29. Inoue S, Shinohara F, Sakai T, et al. Myocarditis and arrhythmia: a clinico-pathological study of conduction system based on serial section in 65 cases. Jpn Circ J 1989;53:49–57.
30. Delacretaz E, Stevenson WG, Winters GL, et al. Ablation of ventricular tachycardia with a saline-cooled radiofrequency catheter: anatomic and histologic characteristics of the lesions in humans. J Cardiovasc Electrophysiol 1999;10:860–865.
31. Woo MA, Stevenson WG, Moser DK, et al. Complex heart rate variability and serum norepinephrine levels in patients with advanced heart failure. J Am Coll Cardiol 1994;23:565–569.
32. Tygesen H, Rundqvist B, Waagstein F, et al. Heart rate variability measurement correlates with cardiac norepinephrine spillover in congestive heart failure. Am J Cardiol 2001;87:1308–1311.
33. Hasking GJ, Esler MD, Jennings GL, et al. Norepinephrine spillover to plasma in patients with congestive heart failure: evidence of increased overall and cardiorenal sympathetic nervous activity. Circulation 1986;73:615–621.
34. Cohn JN, Johnson GR, Shabetai R, et al. Ejection fraction, peak exercise oxygen consumption, cardiothoracic ratio, ventricular arrhythmias, and plasma norepinephrine as determinants of prognosis in heart failure. The V-HeFT VA Cooperative Studies Group. Circulation 1993;87:VI5–V16.
35. Malik M. Heart rate variability. In: Zipes DP, Jalife J, eds. Car-

diac Electrophysiology: From Cell to Bedside. 3rd ed. Philadelphia: W.B. Saunders Co.; 2000:753–762.
36. Fauchier L, Babuty D, Cosnay P, et al. Heart rate variability in idiopathic dilated cardiomyopathy: characteristics and prognostic value. J Am Coll Cardiol 1997;30:1009–1014.
37. Ho KK, Moody GB, Peng CK, et al. Predicting survival in heart failure case and control subjects by use of fully automated methods for deriving nonlinear and conventional indices of heart rate dynamics. Circulation 1997;96:842–848.
38. Uretsky BF, Thygesen K, Armstrong PW, et al. Acute coronary findings at autopsy in heart failure patients with sudden death: results from the Assessment of Treatment with Lisinopril and Survival (ATLAS) trial. Circulation 2000;102:611–616.
39. Stevenson WG, Stevenson LW, Middlekauff HR, et al. Sudden death prevention in patients with advanced ventricular dysfunction. Circulation 1993;88:2953–2961.
40. Adamson PB, Vanoli E. Early autonomic and repolarization abnormalities contribute to lethal arrhythmias in chronic ischemic heart failure: characteristics of a novel heart failure model in dogs with postmyocardial infarction left ventricular dysfunction. J Am Coll Cardiol 2001;37:1741–1748.
41. Dekker LR, Rademaker H, Vermeulen JT, et al. Cellular uncoupling during ischemia in hypertrophied and failing rabbit ventricular myocardium: effects of preconditioning. Circulation 1998;97:1724–1730.
42. Dries DL, Domanski MJ, Waclawiw MA, et al. Effect of antithrombotic therapy on risk of sudden coronary death in patients with congestive heart failure. Am J Cardiol 1997;79:909–913.
43. The Cardiac Insufficiency Bisoprolol Study II (CIBIS-II): a randomised trial. Lancet 1999;353:9–13.
44. Teerlink JR, Massie BM. Beta-adrenergic blocker mortality trials in congestive heart failure. Am J Cardiol 1999;84:94R–102R.
45. Kendall MJ, Lynch KP, Hjalmarson A, et al. Beta-blockers and sudden cardiac death. Ann Intern Med 1995; 123:358–367.
46. Gettes LS. Electrolyte abnormalities underlying lethal and ventricular arrhythmias. Circulation 1992;85:I70–I76.

47. Packer M, Lee WH. Provocation of hyper- and hypokalemic sudden death during treatment with and withdrawal of converting-enzyme inhibition in severe chronic congestive heart failure. Am J Cardiol 1986;57:347–348.
48. Pratt CM, Greenway PS, Schoenfeld MH, et al. Exploration of the precision of classifying sudden cardiac death: implications for the interpretation of clinical trials. Circulation 1996; 93:519–524.
49. Stevenson WG, Sweeney MO. Arrhythmias and sudden death in heart failure. Jpn Circ J 1997;61:727–740.
50. Faggiano P, d'Aloia A, Gualeni A, et al. Mechanisms and immediate outcome of in-hospital cardiac arrest in patients with advanced heart failure secondary to ischemic or idiopathic dilated cardiomyopathy. Am J Cardiol 2001;87:655–657, A10–11.
51. Stellbrink C, Auricchio A, Diem B, et al. Potential benefit of biventricular pacing in patients with congestive heart failure and ventricular tachyarrhythmia. Am J Cardiol 1999;83: 143D–150D.
52. Farwell D, Patel NR, Hall A, et al. How many people with heart failure are appropriate for biventricular resynchronization? Eur Heart J 2000;21:1246–1250.
53. Schoeller R, Andresen D, Buttner P, et al. First- or second-degree atrioventricular block as a risk factor in idiopathic dilated cardiomyopathy. Am J Cardiol 1993;71:720–726.
54. Grubman EM, Pavri BB, Shipman T, et al. Cardiac death and stored electrograms in patients with third-generation implantable cardioverter-defibrillators. J Am Coll Cardiol 1998; 32:1056–1062.
55. Effect of enalapril on survival in patients with reduced left ventricular ejection fractions and congestive heart failure. The SOLVD Investigators. N Engl J Med 1991;325: 293–302.
56. Effect of metoprolol CR/XL in chronic heart failure: metoprolol CR/XL Randomised Intervention Trial in Congestive Heart Failure (MERIT-HF). Lancet 1999;353:2001–2007.
57. Effects of enalapril on mortality in severe congestive heart failure. Results of the Cooperative North Scandinavian Enalapril Survival Study (CONSENSUS). The CONSENSUS Trial Study Group. N Engl J Med 1987;316:1429–1435.
58. Nagele H, Rodiger W. Sudden death and tailored medical ther-

apy in elective candidates for heart transplantation. J Heart Lung Transplant 1999;18:869–876.
59. Uretsky BF, Sheahan RG. Primary prevention of sudden cardiac death in heart failure: will the solution be shocking? J Am Coll Cardiol 1997;30:1589–1597.
60. Cohn JN, Goldstein SO, Greenberg BH, et al. A dose-dependent increase in mortality with vesnarinone among patients with severe heart failure. Vesnarinone Trial Investigators. N Engl J Med 1998;339:1810–1816.
61. Pitt B, Poole-Wilson PA, Segal R, et al. Effect of losartan compared with captopril on mortality in patients with symptomatic heart failure: randomised trial: the Losartan Heart Failure Survival Study ELITE II. Lancet 2000; 355:1582–1587.
62. Teerlink JR, Jalaluddin M, Anderson S, et al. Ambulatory ventricular arrhythmias in patients with heart failure do not specifically predict an increased risk of sudden death. PROMISE (Prospective Randomized Milrinone Survival Evaluation) Investigators. Circulation 2000;101:40–46.
63. Fonarow GC, Chelimsky-Fallick C, Stevenson LW, et al. Effect of direct vasodilation with hydralazine versus angiotensin-converting enzyme inhibition with captopril on mortality in advanced heart failure: the Hy-C trial. J Am Coll Cardiol 1992; 19:842–850.
64. Domanski MJ, Exner DV, Borkowf CB, et al. Effect of angiotensin-converting enzyme inhibition on sudden cardiac death in patients following acute myocardial infarction: a meta-analysis of randomized clinical trials. J Am Coll Cardiol 1999;33:598–604.
65. Maisel WH, Stevenson WG. Sudden death and the electrophysiological effects of angiotensin-converting enzyme inhibitors. J Card Fail 2000;6: 80–82.
66. Krumholz HM, Baker DW, Ashton CM, et al. Evaluating quality of care for patients with heart failure. Circulation 2000; 101:E122-E140.
67. De Sutter J, Tavernier R, De Buyzere M, et al. Lipid-lowering drugs and recurrences of life-threatening ventricular arrhythmias in high-risk patients. J Am Coll Cardiol 2000;36:766–772.
68. Exner DV, Reiffel JA, Epstein AE, et al. Beta-blocker use and

survival in patients with ventricular fibrillation or symptomatic ventricular tachycardia: the Antiarrhythmics Versus Implantable Defibrillators (AVID) trial. J Am Coll Cardiol 1999;34:325–333.
69. Kennedy HL, Brooks MM, Barker AH, et al. Beta-blocker therapy in the Cardiac Arrhythmia Suppression Trial. CAST Investigators. Am J Cardiol 1994;74:674–680.
70. Exner DV, Dries DL, Waclawiw MA, et al. Beta-adrenergic blocking agent use and mortality in patients with asymptomatic and symptomatic left ventricular systolic dysfunction: a post hoc analysis of the Studies of Left Ventricular Dysfunction. J Am Coll Cardiol 1999;33:916–923.
71. Khand AU, Rankin AC, Kaye GC, et al. Systematic review of the management of atrial fibrillation in patients with heart failure. Eur Heart J 2000;21:614–632.
72. Ravid S, Podrid PJ, Lampert S, et al. Congestive heart failure induced by six of the newer antiarrhythmic drugs. J Am Coll Cardiol 1989;14:1326–1330.
73. Stevenson WG. Mechanisms and management of arrhythmias in heart failure. Curr Opin Cardiol 1995;10:274–281.
74. Flaker GC, Blackshear JL, McBride R, et al. Antiarrhythmic drug therapy and cardiac mortality in atrial fibrillation. The Stroke Prevention in Atrial Fibrillation Investigators. J Am Coll Cardiol 1992;20:527–532.
75. Stevenson WG, Stevenson LW, Middlekauff HR, et al. Improving survival for patients with atrial fibrillation and advanced heart failure. J Am Coll Cardiol 1996;28:1458–1463. [Published erratum appears in J Am Coll Cardiol 1997 Dec; 30(7):1902.]
76. Kuck KH, Cappato R, Siebels J, et al. Randomized comparison of antiarrhythmic drug therapy with implantable defibrillators in patients resuscitated from cardiac arrest: the Cardiac Arrest Study Hamburg (CASH). Circulation 2000;102:748– 754.
77. Nul DR, Doval HC, Grancelli HO, et al. Heart rate is a marker of amiodarone mortality reduction in severe heart failure. The GESICA-GEMA Investigators. Grupo de Estudio de la Sobrevida en la Insuficiencia Cardiaca en Argentina-Grupo de Estudios Multicentricos en Argentina. J Am Coll Cardiol 1997; 29:1199–1205.

78. Singh SN, Fletcher RD, Fisher SG, et al. Amiodarone in patients with congestive heart failure and asymptomatic ventricular arrhythmia. Survival Trial of Antiarrhythmic Therapy in Congestive Heart Failure [see comments]. N Engl J Med 1995;333:77–82.
79. Massie BM, Shah NB, Pitt B, et al. Importance of assessing changes in ventricular response to atrial fibrillation during evaluation of new heart failure therapies: experience from trials of flosequinan. Am Heart J 1996;132:130–136.
80. Effect of prophylactic amiodarone on mortality after acute myocardial infarction and in congestive heart failure: meta-analysis of individual data from 6500 patients in randomised trials. Amiodarone Trials Meta-Analysis Investigators [see comments]. Lancet 1997;350:1417–1424.
81. Massie BM, Fisher SG, Radford M, et al. Effect of amiodarone on clinical status and left ventricular function in patients with congestive heart failure. CHF-STAT Investigators. Circulation 1996;93:2128–2134. [Published erratum appears in Circulation 1996 Nov 15;94(10):2668.]
82. Nagatsu M, Spinale FG, Koide M, et al. Bradycardia and the role of beta-blockade in the amelioration of left ventricular dysfunction. Circulation 2000;101:653–659.
83. Stevenson WG, Ellison KG, et al. Management of arrhythmias in heart failure. Cardiol Rev 2002;10(1):8–14.
84. Weinfeld MS, Drazner MH, Stevenson WG, et al. Early outcome of initiating amiodarone for atrial fibrillation in advanced heart failure. J Heart Lung Transplant 2000;19:638– 643.
85. Gottlieb SS, Riggio DW, Lauria S, et al. High-dose oral amiodarone loading exerts important hemodynamic actions in patients with congestive heart failure. J Am Coll Cardiol 1994; 23:560–564.
86. Dusman RE, Stanton MS, Miles WM, et al. Clinical features of amiodarone-induced pulmonary toxicity. Circulation 1990; 82:51–59.
87. Singh SN, Fisher SG, Deedwania PC, et al. Pulmonary effect of amiodarone in patients with heart failure. The Congestive Heart Failure-Survival Trial of Antiarrhythmic Therapy (CHF-STAT) Investigators (Veterans Affairs Cooperative Study No. 320). J Am Coll Cardiol 1997;30:514–517.

88. Siniakowicz RM, Narula D, Suster B, et al. Diagnosis of amiodarone pulmonary toxicity with high-resolution computerized tomographic scan. J Cardiovasc Electrophysiol 2001;12: 431–436.
89. Loh KC. Amiodarone-induced thyroid disorders: a clinical review. Postgrad Med J 2000;76:133–140.
90. Doval HC, Nul DR, Grancelli HO, et al. Randomised trial of low-dose amiodarone in severe congestive heart failure. Grupo de Estudio de la Sobrevida en la Insuficiencia Cardiaca en Argentina (GESICA) [see comments]. Lancet 1994;344:493–498.
91. Pratt CM, Camm AJ, Cooper W, et al. Mortality in the Survival With ORal D-sotalol (SWORD) trial: why did patients die? Am J Cardiol 1998;81:869–876.
92. Roy D, Talajic M, Dorian P, et al. Amiodarone to prevent recurrence of atrial fibrillation. Canadian Trial of Atrial Fibrillation Investigators. N Engl J Med 2000;342:913–920.
93. A comparison of antiarrhythmic-drug therapy with implantable defibrillators in patients resuscitated from near-fatal ventricular arrhythmias. The Antiarrhythmics Versus Implantable Defibrillators (AVID) Investigators. N Engl J Med 1997;337: 1576–1583.
94. Connolly SJ, Gent M, Roberts RS, et al. Canadian implantable defibrillator study (CIDS): a randomized trial of the implantable cardioverter defibrillator against amiodarone. Circulation 2000;101:1297–1302.
95. Sheldon R, Connolly S, Krahn A, et al. Identification of patients most likely to benefit from implantable cardioverter-defibrillator therapy: the Canadian Implantable Defibrillator Study [see comments]. Circulation 2000;101:1660–1664.
96. Connolly SJ, Hallstrom AP, Cappato R, et al. Meta-analysis of the implantable cardioverter defibrillator secondary prevention trials. AVID, CASH and CIDS studies. Antiarrhythmics vs Implantable Defibrillator study. Cardiac Arrest Study Hamburg. Canadian Implantable Defibrillator Study. Eur Heart J 2000;21:2071–2078.
97. Domanski MJ, Sakseena S, Epstein AE, et al. Relative effectiveness of the implantable cardioverter-defibrillator and antiarrhythmic drugs in patients with varying degrees of left

ventricular dysfunction who have survived malignant ventricular arrhythmias. AVID Investigators. Antiarrhythmics Versus Implantable Defibrillators. J Am Coll Cardiol 1999; 34:1090–1095.
98. Sweeney MO, Ruskin JN, Garan H, et al. Influence of the implantable cardioverter/defibrillator on sudden death and total mortality in patients evaluated for cardiac transplantation. Circulation 1995;92:3273–3281.
99. Moss AJ. Implantable cardioverter defibrillator therapy: the sickest patients benefit the most [editorial; comment]. Circulation 2000;101:1638–1640.
100. Bocker D, Bansch D, Heinecke A, et al. Potential benefit from implantable cardioverter-defibrillator therapy in patients with and without heart failure. Circulation 1998;98:1636–1643.
101. Juralti NM, Niebauer ML, Al-Khadra AS, et al. Mortality in octogenarians after implantation of implantable cardioverter-defibrillators: when is too old? J Am Coll Cardiol 2000;35 (suppl A):136.
102. Mecca A, Barakat T, Guo H, et al. Implantable cardioverter defibrillator therapy for patients with life-threatening ventricular arrhythmias and severe heart failure. Am J Cardiol 2000;86:875–877.
103. Saxon LA, Wiener I, DeLurgio DB, et al. Implantable defibrillators for high-risk patients with heart failure who are awaiting cardiac transplantation. Am Heart J 1995;130:501–506.
104. Best PJ, Hayes DL, Stanton MS. The potential usage of dual chamber pacing in patients with implantable cardioverter defibrillators. Pacing Clin Electrophysiol 1999;22:79–85.
105. Grines CL, Bashore TM, Boudoulas H, et al. Functional abnormalities in isolated left bundle branch block: the effect of interventricular asynchrony. Circulation 1989;79:845–853.
106. Nielsen JC, Bottcher M, Nielsen TT, et al. Regional myocardial blood flow in patients with sick sinus syndrome randomized to long-term single chamber atrial or dual chamber pacing: effect of pacing mode and rate. J Am Coll Cardiol 2000;35:1453–1461.
107. Tse HF, Lau CP. Long-term effect of right ventricular pacing

on myocardial perfusion and function. J Am Coll Cardiol 1997;29:744–749.
108. Rosenqvist M, Beyer T, Block M, et al. Adverse events with transvenous implantable cardioverter-defibrillators: a prospective multicenter study. European 7219 Jewel ICD investigators. Circulation 1998;98:663–670. [Published erratum appears in Circulation 1998 Dec 8;98(23):2647.]
109. Spotnitz HM. Does ventricular fibrillation cause myocardial stunning during defibrillator implantation? J Card Surg 1993;8:249–256.
110. Michaud GF, Pelosi F Jr, Noble MD, et al. A randomized trial comparing heparin initiation 6 h or 24 h after pacemaker or defibrillator implantation. J Am Coll Cardiol 2000;35:1915–1918.
111. Spinler SA, Nawarskas JJ, Foote EF, et al. Clinical presentation and analysis of risk factors for infectious complications of implantable cardioverter-defibrillator implantations at a university medical center. Clin Infect Dis 1998;26:1111–1116.
112. Smith PN, Vidaillet HJ, Hayes JJ, et al. Infections with nonthoracotomy implantable cardioverter defibrillators: can these be prevented? Endotak Lead Clinical Investigators. Pacing Clin Electrophysiol 1998;21:42–55.
113. Pires LA, Lehmann MH, Steinman RT, et al. Sudden death in implantable cardioverter-defibrillator recipients: clinical context, arrhythmic events and device responses [see comments]. J Am Coll Cardiol 1999;33:24–32.
114. Villacastin J, Almendral J, Arenal A, et al. Incidence and clinical significance of multiple consecutive, appropriate, high-energy discharges in patients with implanted cardioverter-defibrillators. Circulation 1996;93:753–762.
115. Exner DV, Pinski SL, Wyse DG, et al. Electrical storm presages nonsudden death: the Antiarrhythmics Versus Implantable Defibrillators (AVID) Trial. Circulation 2001;103:2066–2071.
116. Thomas SA, Friedmann E, Kelley FJ. Living with an implantable cardioverter-defibrillator: a review of the current literature related to psychosocial factors. AACN Clin Issues 2001;12:156–163.

117. Sears SF, Todaro JF, Urizar G, et al. Assessing the psychosocial impact of the ICD: a national survey of implantable cardioverter defibrillator health care providers. Pacing Clin Electrophysiol 2000;23:939–945.
118. Dunbar SB, Kimble LP, Jenkins LS, et al. Association of mood disturbance and arrhythmia events in patients after cardioverter defibrillator implantation. Depress Anxiety 1999; 9:163–168.
119. Heller SS, Ormont MA, Lidagoster L, et al. Psychosocial outcome after ICD implantation: a current perspective. Pacing Clin Electrophysiol 1998;21:1207–1215.
120. Fricchione GL, Vlay LC, Vlay SC. Cardiac psychiatry and the management of malignant ventricular arrhythmias with the internal cardioverter-defibrillator. Am Heart J 1994;128:1050–1059.
121. Ruppel R, Schluter CA, Boczor S, et al. Ventricular tachycardia during follow-up in patients resuscitated from ventricular fibrillation: experience from stored electrograms of implantable cardioverter-defibrillators. J Am Coll Cardiol 1998;32:1724–1730.
122. Wang YS, Scheinman MM, Chien WW, et al. Patients with supraventricular tachycardia presenting with aborted sudden death: incidence, mechanism and long-term follow-up [see comments]. J Am Coll Cardiol 1991;18:1711–1719.
123. Hays LJ, Lerman BB, DiMarco JP. Nonventricular arrhythmias as precursors of ventricular fibrillation in patients with out-of-hospital cardiac arrest. Am Heart J 1989;118:53–57.
124. Hallstrom AP, McAnulty JH, Wilkoff BL, et al. Patients at lower risk of arrhythmia recurrence: a subgroup in whom implantable defibrillators may not offer benefit. Antiarrhythmics Versus Implantable Defibrillators (AVID) Trial Investigators. J Am Coll Cardiol 2001;37:1093–1099.
125. The AVID Investigators. Causes of death in the Antiarrhythmics Versus Implantable Defibrillators (AVID) trial. J Am Coll Cardiol 1999;34:1552–1559.
126. Brugada P, Talajic M, Smeets J, et al. The value of the clinical history to assess prognosis of patients with ventricular tachycardia or ventricular fibrillation after myocardial infarction. Eur Heart J 1989;10:747–752.

127. Willems AR, Tijssen JG, van Capelle FJ, et al. Determinants of prognosis in symptomatic ventricular tachycardia or ventricular fibrillation late after myocardial infarction. The Dutch Ventricular Tachycardia Study Group of the Interuniversity Cardiology Institute of The Netherlands [see comments]. J Am Coll Cardiol 1990;16:521–530.
128. Anderson JL, Hallstrom AP, Epstein AE, et al. Design and results of the Antiarrhythmics Versus Implantable Defibrillators (AVID) registry. The AVID Investigators. Circulation 1999;99:1692–1699.
129. Epstein AE, Powell J, Yao Q, et al. In-hospital versus out-of-hospital presentation of life-threatening ventricular arrhythmias predicts survival: results from the AVID Registry. Antiarrhythmics Versus Implantable Defibrillators. J Am Coll Cardiol 1999;34:1111–1116.
130. Natale A, Sra J, Axtell K, et al. Ventricular fibrillation and polymorphic ventricular tachycardia with critical coronary artery stenosis: does bypass surgery suffice? J Cardiovasc Electrophysiol 1994;5:988–994.
131. Volpi A, Cavalli A, Turato R, et al. Incidence and short-term prognosis of late sustained ventricular tachycardia after myocardial infarction: results of the Gruppo Italiano per lo Studio della Sopravvivenza nell'Infarto Miocardico (GISSI-3) Data Base. Am Heart J 2001;142:87–92.
132. Brugada P, Brugada J, Mont L, et al. A new approach to the differential diagnosis of a regular tachycardia with a wide QRS complex. Circulation 1991;83:1649–1659.
133. Drew BJ, Scheinman MM. ECG criteria to distinguish between aberrantly conducted supraventricular tachycardia and ventricular tachycardia: practical aspects for the immediate care setting. Pacing Clin Electrophysiol 1995;18:2194–2208.
134. Akhtar M, Shenasa M, Jazayeri M, et al. Wide QRS complex tachycardia. Reappraisal of a common clinical problem. Ann Intern Med 1988;109:905–912.
135. Oreto G, Smeets JL, Rodriguez LM, et al. Wide complex tachycardia with atrioventricular dissociation and QRS morphology identical to that of sinus rhythm: a manifestation of bundle branch reentry. Heart 1996;76:541–547.

136. Blanck Z, Dhala A, Deshpande S, et al. Bundle branch reentrant ventricular tachycardia: cumulative experience in 48 patients. J Cardiovasc Electrophysiol 1993; 4:253–262.
137. Peters S, Peters H, Thierfelder L. Heart failure in arrhythmogenic right ventricular dysplasia-cardiomyopathy. Int J Cardiol 1999;71:251–256.
138. Shinbane JS, Wood MA, Jensen DN, et al. Tachycardia-induced cardiomyopathy: a review of animal models and clinical studies. J Am Coll Cardiol 1997;29:709–715.
139. Jaggarao NS, Nanda AS, Daubert JP. Ventricular tachycardia-induced cardiomyopathy: improvement with radiofrequency ablation. Pacing Clin Electrophysiol 1996;19:505– 508.
140. Singh B, Kaul U, Talwar KK, et al. Reversibility of "tachycardia-induced cardiomyopathy" following the cure of idiopathic left ventricular tachycardia using radiofrequency energy. Pacing Clin Electrophysiol 1996;19:1391–1392.
141. Vijgen J, Hill P, Biblo LA, et al. Tachycardia-induced cardiomyopathy secondary to right ventricular outflow tract ventricular tachycardia: improvement of left ventricular systolic function after radiofrequency catheter ablation of the arrhythmia. J Cardiovasc Electrophysiol 1997;8:445–450.
142. Lerman BB, Stein KM, Markowitz SM, et al. Ventricular arrhythmias in normal hearts. Cardiol Clin 2000;18:265–291, vii.
143. Rodriguez LM, Smeets JL, Timmermans C, et al. Predictors for successful ablation of right- and left-sided idiopathic ventricular tachycardia. Am J Cardiol 1997;79:309–314.
144. Woelfel A, Wohns DH, Foster JR. Implications of sustained monomorphic ventricular tachycardia associated with myocardial injury. Ann Intern Med 1990;112:141–143.
145. Soejima K, Suzuki M, Maisel WH, et al. Catheter ablation in patients with multiple and unstable ventricular tachycardias after myocardial infarction: short ablation lines guided by reentry circuit isthmuses and sinus rhythm mapping. Circulation 2001;104:664–669.
146. Capucci A, Aschieri D, Villani GQ. The role of EP-guided therapy in ventricular arrhythmias: beta-blockers, sotalol, and ICDs. J Interv Card Electrophysiol 2000;4(suppl 1):57– 63.
147. Raitt MH, Renfroe EG, Epstein AE, et al. "Stable" ventricular

tachycardia is not a benign rhythm: insights from the Antiarrhythmics Versus Implantable Defibrillators (AVID) registry. Circulation 2001;103:244–252.
148. Passman R, Kadish A. Polymorphic ventricular tachycardia, long Q-T syndrome, and torsades de pointes. Med Clin North Am 2001;85:321–341.
149. Kowey PR, VanderLugt JT, Luderer JR. Safety and risk/benefit analysis of ibutilide for acute conversion of atrial fibrillation/flutter. Am J Cardiol 1996;78:46–52.
150. Mazur A, Anderson ME, Bonney S, et al. Pause-dependent polymorphic ventricular tachycardia during long-term treatment with dofetilide: a placebo-controlled, implantable cardioverter-defibrillator-based evaluation. J Am Coll Cardiol 2001;37:1100–1105.
151. Maor N, Weiss D, Lorber A. Torsade de pointes complicating atrioventricular block: report of two cases. Int J Cardiol 1987;14:235–238.
152. Viskin S, Glikson M, Fish R, et al. Rate smoothing with cardiac pacing for preventing torsade de pointes. Am J Cardiol 2000;86:K111-K115.
153. Merrill LC website. Guidant Corp. more MADIT II data. Merrill Lynch Comment. November 28, 2001.
154. Singh SN, Fisher SG, Carson PE, et al. Prevalence and significance of nonsustained ventricular tachycardia in patients with premature ventricular contractions and heart failure treated with vasodilator therapy. Department of Veterans Affairs CHF STAT Investigators. J Am Coll Cardiol 1998;32:942–947.
155. Doval HC, Nul DR, Grancelli HO, et al. Nonsustained ventricular tachycardia in severe heart failure: independent marker of increased mortality due to sudden death. GESICA-GEMA Investigators. Circulation 1996;94: 3198–3203.
156. Davies SW, John LM, Wedzicha JA, et al. Overnight studies in severe chronic left heart failure: arrhythmias and oxygen desaturation. Br Heart J 1991;65:77–83.
157. Javaheri S. Effects of continuous positive airway pressure on sleep apnea and ventricular irritability in patients with heart failure. Circulation 2000;101:392–397.
158. Javaheri S, Parker TJ, Liming JD, et al. Sleep apnea in 81 am-

bulatory male patients with stable heart failure: types and their prevalences, consequences, and presentations [see comments]. Circulation 1998;97:2154–2159.
159. Javaheri S, Corbett WS. Association of low $PaCO_2$ with central sleep apnea and ventricular arrhythmias in ambulatory patients with stable heart failure. Ann Intern Med 1998;128: 204–207.
160. Buxton AE, Lee KL, Fisher JD, et al. A randomized study of the prevention of sudden death in patients with coronary artery disease. Multicenter Unsustained Tachycardia Trial Investigators. N Engl J Med 1999;341:1882– 1890. [Published erratum appears in N Engl J Med 2000 27;342(17):1300.]
161. Moss AJ, Hall WJ, Cannom DS, et al. Improved survival with an implanted defibrillator in patients with coronary disease at high risk for ventricular arrhythmia. Multicenter Automatic Defibrillator Implantation Trial Investigators [see comments]. N Engl J Med 1996;335:1933–1940.
162. Bigger JT Jr, Whang W, Rottman JN, et al. Mechanisms of death in the CABG Patch trial: a randomized trial of implantable cardiac defibrillator prophylaxis in patients at high risk of death after coronary artery bypass graft surgery. Circulation 1999;99:1416–1421.
163. Buxton AE, Lee KL, DiCarlo L, et al. Electrophysiologic testing to identify patients with coronary artery disease who are at risk for sudden death. Multicenter Unsustained Tachycardia Trial Investigators. N Engl J Med 2000;342:1937–1945.
164. Hammill SC, Trusty JM, Wood DL, et al. Influence of ventricular function and presence or absence of coronary artery disease on results of electrophysiologic testing for asymptomatic nonsustained ventricular tachycardia. Am J Cardiol 1990;65:722–728.
165. Lindsay BD, Osborn JL, Schechtman KB, et al. Prospective detection of vulnerability to sustained ventricular tachycardia in patients awaiting cardiac transplantation. Am J Cardiol 1992;69:619–624.
166. Das SK, Morady F, DiCarlo L Jr, et al. Prognostic usefulness of programmed ventricular stimulation in idiopathic dilated cardiomyopathy without symptomatic ventricular arrhythmias. Am J Cardiol 1986;58:998–1000.

167. Meinertz T, Treese N, Kasper W, et al. Determinants of prognosis in idiopathic dilated cardiomyopathy as determined by programmed electrical stimulation. Am J Cardiol 1985; 56:337–341.
168. Poll DS, Marchlinski FE, Buxton AE, et al. Usefulness of programmed stimulation in idiopathic dilated cardiomyopathy. Am J Cardiol 1986;58:992–997.
169. Strickberger A, et al. AMIOVIRT Multicenter Randomized Trial Comparing Amiodarone to ICD in patients with nonischemic dilated cardiomyopathy and nonsustained ventricular tachycardia (submitted—personal communication), 2001.
170. Connolly SJ. Meta-analysis of antiarrhythmic drug trials. Am J Cardiol 1999;84:90R-93R.
171. Barold HS, Hesselson AB, Jollis J, et al. Concealed mechanical bradycardia: an indication for permanent pacemaker implantation. Pacing Clin Electrophysiol 1998;21:2007–2008.
172. Huikuri HV, Makikallio T, Airaksinen KE, et al. Measurement of heart rate variability: a clinical tool or a research toy? J Am Coll Cardiol 1999;34:1878–1883.
173. Myers G, Workman M, Birkett C, et al. Problems in measuring heart rate variability of patients with congestive heart failure. J Electrocardiol 1992;25:214–219.
174. El-Omar M, Kardos A, Casadei B. Mechanisms of respiratory sinus arrhythmia in patients with mild heart failure. Am J Physiol Heart Circ Physiol 2001;280:H125–H131.
175. Casolo GC, Stroder P, Sulla A, et al. Heart rate variability and functional severity of congestive heart failure secondary to coronary artery disease. Eur Heart J 1995;16:360–367.
176. Fei L, Keeling PJ, Gill JS, et al. Heart rate variability and its relation to ventricular arrhythmias in congestive heart failure. Br Heart J 1994;71:322–328.
177. Hoffmann J, Grimm W, Menz V, et al. Heart rate variability and baroreflex sensitivity in idiopathic dilated cardiomyopathy. Heart 2000;83:531–538.
178. Szabo BM, van Veldhuisen DJ, van der Veer N, et al. Prognostic value of heart rate variability in chronic congestive heart failure secondary to idiopathic or ischemic dilated cardiomyopathy. Am J Cardiol 1997;79:978–980.

179. Szabo BM, van Veldhuisen DJ, Brouwer J, et al. Relation between severity of disease and impairment of heart rate variability parameters in patients with chronic congestive heart failure secondary to coronary artery disease. Am J Cardiol 1995;76:713–716.
180. Jiang W, Hathaway WR, McNulty S, et al. Ability of heart rate variability to predict prognosis in patients with advanced congestive heart failure. Am J Cardiol 1997;80:808– 811.
181. Makikallio TH, Huikuri HV, Hintze U, et al. Fractal analysis and time- and frequency-domain measures of heart rate variability as predictors of mortality in patients with heart failure. Am J Cardiol 2001;87:178–182.
182. Gregoratos G, Cheitlin MD, Conill A, et al. ACC/AHA guidelines for implantation of cardiac pacemakers and antiarrhythmia devices: executive summary: a report of the American College of Cardiology/American Heart Association Task Force on Practice Guidelines (Committee on Pacemaker Implantation). Circulation 1998;97:1325–1335.
183. Batchvarov V, Malik M. Measurement and interpretation of QT dispersion. Prog Cardiovasc Dis 2000;42:325–344.
184. Brendorp B, Elming H, Jun L, et al. QT dispersion has no prognostic information for patients with advanced congestive heart failure and reduced left ventricular systolic function. Circulation 2001;103:831–835.
185. Spargias KS, Lindsay SJ, Kawar GI, et al. QT dispersion as a predictor of long-term mortality in patients with acute myocardial infarction and clinical evidence of heart failure. Eur Heart J 1999;20:1158–1165.
186. Berger RD, Kasper EK, Baughman KL, et al. Beat-to-beat QT interval variability: novel evidence for repolarization lability in ischemic and nonischemic dilated cardiomyopathy. Circulation 1997;96:1557–1565.
187. Atiga WL, Calkins H, Lawrence JH, et al. Beat-to-beat repolarization lability identifies patients at risk for sudden cardiac death. J Cardiovasc Electrophysiol 1998;9:899–908.
188. Murda'h MA, McKenna WJ, Camm AJ. Repolarization alternans: techniques, mechanisms, and cardiac vulnerability. Pacing Clin Electrophysiol 1997;20:2641–2657.

189. Qu Z, Garfinkel A, Chen PS, et al. Mechanisms of discordant alternans and induction of reentry in simulated cardiac tissue. Circulation 2000;102:1664–1670.
190. Rosenbaum DS. T wave alternans: a mechanism of arrhythmogenesis comes of age after 100 years. J Cardiovasc Electrophysiol 2001;12:207–209.
191. Turitto G, Caref EB, El-Attar G, et al. Optimal target heart rate for exercise-induced T-wave alternans. Ann Noninvasive Electrocardiol 2001;6:123–128.
192. Gold MR, Bloomfield DM, Anderson KP, et al. A comparison of T-wave alternans, signal-averaged electrocardiography and programmed ventricular stimulation for arrhythmia risk stratification. J Am Coll Cardiol 2000;36:2247–2253.
193. Hennersdorf MG, Perings C, Niebch V, et al. T wave alternans as a risk predictor in patients with cardiomyopathy and mild-to-moderate heart failure. Pacing Clin Electrophysiol 2000;23:1386–1391.
194. Klingenheben T, Zabel M, D'Agostino RB, et al. Predictive value of T-wave alternans for arrhythmic events in patients with congestive heart failure. Lancet 2000;356:651–652.
195. Tapanainen JM, Still AM, Airaksinen KE, et al. Prognostic significance of risk stratifiers of mortality, including T wave alternans, after acute myocardial infarction: results of a prospective follow-up study. J Cardiovasc Electrophysiol 2001; 12:645–652.
196. Adachi K, Ohnishi Y, Shima T, et al. Determinant of microvolt-level T-wave alternans in patients with dilated cardiomyopathy. J Am Coll Cardiol 1999;34:374–380.
197. Rosenbaum DS, Jackson LE, Smith JM, et al. Electrical alternans and vulnerability to ventricular arrhythmias. N Engl J Med 1994;330:235–241.
198. Grimm W, Hoffmann J, Menz V, et al. Relation between microvolt level T wave alternans and other potential noninvasive predictors of arrhythmic risk in the Marburg Cardiomyopathy Study. Pacing Clin Electrophysiol 2000;23:1960–1964.
199. Kapoor W. Syncope. N Engl J Med 2000;343:1856–1862.
200. Kapoor WN. Evaluation and management of the patient with syncope. JAMA 1992;268:2553–2560.

201. Kapoor WN. Evaluation and outcome of patients with syncope. Medicine 1990;69:160–175.
202. Manolis AS, Linzer M, Salem D, et al. Syncope: current diagnostic evaluation and management. Ann Intern Med 1990; 112:850–863.
203. Fonarow GC, Feliciano Z, Boyle NG, et al. Improved survival in patients with nonischemic advanced heart failure and syncope treated with an implantable cardioverter-defibrillator. Am J Cardiol 2000;85:981–985.
204. Fruhwald FM, Eber B, Schumacher M, et al. Syncope in dilated cardiomyopathy is a predictor of sudden cardiac death. Cardiology 1996;87:177–180.
205. Knight BP, Goyal R, Pelosi F, et al. Outcome of patients with nonischemic dilated cardiomyopathy and unexplained syncope treated with an implantable defibrillator. J Am Coll Cardiol 1999;33:1964–1970.
206. Middlekauff HR, Stevenson WG, Stevenson LW, et al. Syncope in advanced heart failure: high risk of sudden death regardless of origin of syncope. J Am Coll Cardiol 1993;21: 110–116.
207. Atkins D, Hanusa B, Sefcik T, et al. Syncope and orthostatic hypotension. Am J Med 1991;91:179–185.
208. Meyer MD, Handler J. Evaluation of the patient with syncope: an evidence based approach. Emerg Med Clin North Am 1999;17:189–201.
209. Hoefnagels WAJ, Padberg GW, Overweg J, et al. Transient loss of consciousness: the value of the history for distinguishing seizure from syncope. J Neurol 1991;238:39–43.
210. Day SC, Cook EF, Funkenstein H, et al. Evaluation and outcome of emergency room patients with transient loss of consciousness. Am J Med 1982;73:15–23.
211. Georgeson S, Linzer M, Griffith JL, et al. Acute cardiac ischemia in patients with syncope: importance of initial electrocardiogram. J Gen Intern Med 1992;7:379–386.
212. Linzer M, Yang EH, Estes NAM III, et al. Diagnosing syncope part 2: unexplained syncope. Ann Intern Med 1997;127: 76–86.
213. Krahn AD, Klein GJ, Yee R, et al. Use of an extended monitoring strategy in patients with problematic syncope. Circulation 1999;99:406–410.

214. Zipes DP, DiMarco JP, Gillette PC, et al. ACC/AHA guidelines for clinical intracardiac electrophysiological and catheter ablation procedures. Circulation 1995;92:675–691.
215. Fujimura O, Yee R, Klein GJ, et al. The diagnostic sensitivity of electrophysiologic testing in patients with syncope caused by transient bradycardia. N Engl J Med 1989;321: 1703–1707.
216. Gregoratos G, Cheitlin MD, Conill A, et al. ACC/AHA guidelines for implantation of cardiac pacemakers and antiarrhythmia devices: executive summary. Circulation 1998;97: 1325–1335.
217. Mittal S, Iwai S, Stein KM, et al. Long-term outcome of patients with unexplained syncope treated with an electrophysiologic-guided approach in the implantable cardioverter-defibrillator era. J Am Coll Cardiol 1999;34:1082–1089.
218. Andrews NP, Fogel RI, Pelargonio G, et al. Implantable defibrillator event rates in patients with unexplained syncope and inducible sustained ventricular tachyarrhythmias. J Am Coll Cardiol 1999;34:2023–2030.
219. Middlekauff HR, Stevenson WG, Saxon LA. Prognosis after syncope: impact of left ventricular function. Am Heart J 1993; 125:121–127.
220. Linde-Edelstam C, Gullberg B, Norlander R, et al. Longevity in patients with high degree atrioventricular block paced in the atrial synchronous or the fixed rate ventricular inhibited mode. Pacing Clin Electrophysiol 1992;15:304–313.
221. Connolly SJ, Kerr CR, Gent M, et al. Effects of physiologic pacing versus ventricular pacing on the risk of stroke and death due to cardiovascular causes. Canadian Trial of Physiologic Pacing Investigators. N Engl J Med 2000;342:1385–1391.
222. Nishimura RA, Hayes DL, Holmes DR Jr, et al. Mechanism of hemodynamic improvement by dual-chamber pacing for severe left ventricular dysfunction: an acute Doppler and catheterization hemodynamic study. J Am Coll Cardiol 1995; 25:281–288.
223. Sack S, Franz R, Dagres N, et al. Can right-sided atrioventricular sequential pacing provide benefit for selected patients with severe congestive heart failure? Am J Cardiol 1999;83:124D–129D.

224. Vanderheyden M, Goethals M, Anguera I, et al. Hemodynamic deterioration following radiofrequency ablation of the atrioventricular conduction system. Pacing Clin Electrophysiol 1997;20:2422–2428.
225. Nielsen JC, Andersen HR, Thomsen PE, et al. Heart failure and echocardiographic changes during long-term follow-up of patients with sick sinus syndrome randomized to single-chamber atrial or ventricular pacing. Circulation 1998;97: 987–995.
226. Blanc JJ, Etienne Y, Gilard M, et al. Evaluation of different ventricular pacing sites in patients with severe heart failure: results of an acute hemodynamic study. Circulation 1997;96: 3273–3277.
227. Auricchio A, Salo RW. Acute hemodynamic improvement by pacing in patients with severe congestive heart failure. Pacing Clin Electrophysiol 1997;20:313–324.
228. Twidale N, Manda V, Holliday R, et al. Mitral regurgitation after atrioventricular node catheter ablation for atrial fibrillation and heart failure: acute hemodynamic features [see comments]. Am Heart J 1999;138:1166–1175.
229. Saxon LA, Stevenson WG, Middlekauff HR, et al. Increased risk of progressive hemodynamic deterioration in advanced heart failure patients requiring permanent pacemakers. Am Heart J 1993;125:1306–1310.
230. Saxon LA, Stevenson WG, Middlekauff HR, et al. Predicting death from progressive heart failure secondary to ischemic or idiopathic dilated cardiomyopathy. Am J Cardiol 1993;72: 62–65.
231. Pinski SL, Yao Q, Epstein AE, et al. Determinants of outcome in patients with sustained ventricular tachyarrhythmias: the Antiarrhythmics Versus Implantable Defibrillators (AVID) study registry. Am Heart J 2000;139:804–813.
232. Cazeau S, Leclercq C, Lavergne T, et al. Effects of multisite biventricular pacing in patients with heart failure and intraventricular conduction delay. N Engl J Med 2001;344:873–880.
233. Leclercq C, Cazeau S, Le Breton H, et al. Acute hemodynamic effects of biventricular DDD pacing in patients with end-stage heart failure. J Am Coll Cardiol 1998;32:1825–1831.

234. Kerwin WF, Botvinick EH, O'Connell JW, et al. Ventricular contraction abnormalities in dilated cardiomyopathy: effect of biventricular pacing to correct interventricular dyssynchrony. J Am Coll Cardiol 2000;35:1221–1227.
235. Kass DA, Chen CH, Curry C, et al. Improved left ventricular mechanics from acute VDD pacing in patients with dilated cardiomyopathy and ventricular conduction delay. Circulation 1999;99:1567–1573.
236. Hamdan MH, Zagrodzky JD, Joglar JA, et al. Biventricular pacing decreases sympathetic activity compared with right ventricular pacing in patients with depressed ejection fraction. Circulation 2000;102:1027–1032.
237. Lau CP, Yu CM, Chau E, et al. Reversal of left ventricular remodeling by synchronous biventricular pacing in heart failure. Pacing Clin Electrophysiol 2000;23:1722–1725.
238. Auricchio A, Stellbrink C, Sack S, et al. Long-term benefit as a result of pacing resynchronization in congestive heart failure: results of the Path-CHF trial. Circulation 2000;102: 693A.
239. Daubert JC, Linde C, Cazeau S, et al. Clinical effects of biventricular pacing in patients with severe heart failure and normal sinus rhythm: results from the Multisite Stimulation in Cardiomyopathy-MUSTIC-Group I. Circulation 2000;102: 694A.
240. Reuter S, Garrigue S, Bordachar P, et al. Intermediate-term results of biventricular pacing in heart failure: correlation between clinical and hemodynamic data. Pacing Clin Electrophysiol 2000;23:1713–1717.
241. Higgins SL, Yong P, Scheck D, et al. Biventricular pacing diminishes the need for implantable cardioverter defibrillator therapy. J Am Coll Cardiol 2000;36:824–827.
242. Walker S, Levy TM, Paul VE. Biventricular pacing decreased ventricular arrhythmia. Circulation 2000;102:692A.
243. Abraham WT. Rationale and design of a randomized clinical trial to assess the safety and efficacy of cardiac resynchronization therapy in patients with advanced heart failure: the Multicenter InSync Randomized Clinical Evaluation (MIRACLE). J Card Fail 2000;6:369–380.
244. Mahoney P, Kimmel S, DeNofrio D, et al. Prognostic signifi-

cance of atrial fibrillation in patients at a tertiary medical center referred for heart transplantation because of severe heart failure. Am J Cardiol 1999;83:1544–1547.
245. Dries DL, Exner DV, Gersh BJ, et al. Atrial fibrillation is associated with an increased risk for mortality and heart failure progression in patients with asymptomatic and symptomatic left ventricular systolic dysfunction: a retrospective analysis of the SOLVD trials. Studies of left ventricular dysfunction. J Am Coll Cardiol 1998;32:695–703.
246. Deedwania PC, Singh BN, Ellenbogen K, et al. Spontaneous conversion and maintenance of sinus rhythm by amiodarone in patients with heart failure and atrial fibrillation: observations from the Veterans Affairs Congestive Heart Failure Survival Trial of Antiarrhythmic Therapy (CHF-STAT). The Department of Veterans Affairs CHF-STAT Investigators. Circulation 1998;98:2574–2579.
247. Pedersen OD, Bagger H, Kober L, et al. The occurrence and prognostic significance of atrial fibrillation/flutter following acute myocardial infarction. TRACE Study group. TRAndolapril Cardiac Evaluation. Eur Heart J 1999; 20:748–754.
248. Crijns HJ, Tjeerdsma G, de Kam PJ, et al. Prognostic value of the presence and development of atrial fibrillation in patients with advanced chronic heart failure. Eur Heart J 2000; 21:1238–1245.
249. Kay GN, Ellenbogen KA, Giudici M, et al. The Ablate and Pace Trial: a prospective study of catheter ablation of the AV conduction system and permanent pacemaker implantation for treatment of atrial fibrillation. APT Investigators [see comments]. J Interv Card Electrophysiol 1998;2:121–135.
250. Pardaens K, Van Cleemput J, Vanhaecke J, et al. Atrial fibrillation is associated with a lower exercise capacity in male chronic heart failure patients. Heart 1997;78:564–568.
251. Verma A, Newman D, Geist M, et al. Effects of rhythm regularization and rate control in improving left ventricular function in atrial fibrillation patients undergoing atrioventricular nodal ablation. Can J Cardiol 2001;17:437–445.
252. Carson PE, Johnson GR, Dunkman WB, et al. The influence of atrial fibrillation on prognosis in mild to moderate heart

failure. The V-HeFT Studies. The V-HeFT VA Cooperative Studies Group. Circulation 1993;87:VI102–VI110.
253. Predictors of thromboembolism in atrial fibrillation: Clinical features of patients at risk. Stroke Prevention in Atrial Fibrillation Investigators. Ann Intern Med 1992;116:1–5.
254. Fuster V, Ryden LE, Asinger RW, et al. ACC/AHA/ESC guidelines for the management of patients with atrial fibrillation: executive summary. A Report of the American College of Cardiology/ American Heart Association Task Force on Practice Guidelines and the European Society of Cardiology Committee for Practice Guidelines and Policy Conferences (Committee to Develop Guidelines for the Management of Patients with Atrial Fibrillation): developed in collaboration with the North American Society of Pacing and Electrophysiology. J Am Coll Cardiol 2001;38:1231–1265.
255. Tuinenburg AE, Van Gelder IC, Van Den Berg MP, et al. Lack of prevention of heart failure by serial electrical cardioversion in patients with persistent atrial fibrillation. Heart 1999; 82:486–493.
256. Middlekauff HR, Wiener I, Saxon LA, et al. Low-dose amiodarone for atrial fibrillation: time for a prospective study? Ann Intern Med 1992;116:1017–1020.
257. Grogan M, Smith HC, Gersh BJ, et al. Left ventricular dysfunction due to atrial fibrillation in patients initially believed to have idiopathic dilated cardiomyopathy. Am J Cardiol 1992;69:1570–3173.
258. Ueng KC, Tsai TP, Tsai CF, et al. Acute and long-term effects of atrioventricular junction ablation and VVIR pacemaker in symptomatic patients with chronic lone atrial fibrillation and normal ventricular response. J Cardiovasc Electrophysiol 2001;12:303–309.
259. Heywood JT. Calcium channel blockers for heart rate control in atrial fibrillation complicated by congestive heart failure. Can J Cardiol 1995;11:823–826.
260. Brown CS, Mills RM Jr, Conti JB, et al. Clinical improvement after atrioventricular nodal ablation for atrial fibrillation does not correlate with improved ejection fraction. Am J Cardiol 1997;80:1090–1091.

261. Brignole M, Menozzi C, Gianfranchi L, et al. Assessment of atrioventricular junction ablation and VVIR pacemaker versus pharmacological treatment in patients with heart failure and chronic atrial fibrillation: a randomized, controlled study. Circulation 1998;98:953–960.
262. Proclemer A, Della Bella P, Tondo C, et al. Radiofrequency ablation of atrioventricular junction and pacemaker implantation versus modulation of atrioventricular conduction in drug refractory atrial fibrillation. Am J Cardiol 1999;83: 1437–1442.
263. Fitzpatrick AP, Kourouyan HD, Siu A, et al. Quality of life and outcomes after radiofrequency His-bundle catheter ablation and permanent pacemaker implantation: impact of treatment in paroxysmal and established atrial fibrillation. Am Heart J 1996;131:499–507.
264. Manolis AG, Katsivas AG, Lazaris EE, et al. Ventricular performance and quality of life in patients who underwent radiofrequency AV junction ablation and permanent pacemaker implantation due to medically refractory atrial tachyarrhythmias. J Interv Card Electrophysiol 1998;2:71–76.
265. Levy T, Walker S, Mason M, et al. Importance of rate control or rate regulation for improving exercise capacity and quality of life in patients with permanent atrial fibrillation and normal left ventricular function: a randomized controlled study. Heart 2001;85:171–178.
266. Falk RH. Atrial fibrillation. N Engl J Med 2001;344:1067–1078.
267. Edner M, Caidahl K, Bergfeldt L, et al. Prospective study of left ventricular function after radiofrequency ablation of atrioventricular junction in patients with atrial fibrillation. Br Heart J 1995;74:261–267.
268. Geelen P, Brugada J, Andries E, et al. Ventricular fibrillation and sudden death after radiofrequency catheter ablation of the atrioventricular junction. Pacing Clin Electrophysiol 1997;20:343–348.
269. Corrado G, Sgalambro A, Mantero A, et al. Thromboembolic risk in atrial flutter. The FLASIEC (FLutter Atriale Societa Ialiana di Ecografia Cardiovascolare) multicentre study. Eur Heart J 2001;22:1042–1051.

270. Lanzarotti CJ, Olshansky B. Thromboembolism in chronic atrial flutter: is the risk underestimated? J Am Coll Cardiol 1997;30:1506–1511.
271. Schmidt H, von der Recke G, Illien S, et al. Prevalence of left atrial chamber and appendage thrombi in patients with atrial flutter and its clinical significance. J Am Coll Cardiol 2001;38:778–784.
272. Seidl K, Hauer B, Schwick NG, et al. Risk of thromboembolic events in patients with atrial flutter. Am J Cardiol 1998;82:580–583.
273. Wood KA, Eisenberg SJ, Kalman JM, et al. Risk of thromboembolism in chronic atrial flutter. Am J Cardiol 1997;79:1043–1047.
274. Crijns HJ, Van Gelder IC, Tieleman RG, et al. Long-term outcome of electrical cardioversion in patients with chronic atrial flutter. Heart 1997;77:56–61.
275. Luchsinger JA, Steinberg JS. Resolution of cardiomyopathy after ablation of atrial flutter. J Am Coll Cardiol 1998;32:205–210.
276. Natale A, Newby KH, Pisano E, et al. Prospective randomized comparison of antiarrhythmic therapy versus first-line radiofrequency ablation in patients with atrial flutter. J Am Coll Cardiol 2000;35:1898–1904.
277. Paydak H, Kall JG, Burke MC, et al. Atrial fibrillation after radiofrequency ablation of type I atrial flutter: time to onset, determinants, and clinical course. Circulation 1998;98:315–322.
278. Huang DT, Monahan KM, Zimetbaum P, et al. Hybrid pharmacologic and ablative therapy: a novel and effective approach for the management of atrial fibrillation. J Cardiovasc Electrophysiol 1998;9:462–469.

Index

Amiodarone, 4, 13–15, 36, 48, 50–52
    atrial fibrillation and flutter, 70–72
    bradycardia and, 15, 61
    hyper- and hypothyroidism, 14
    ICDs, 15, 50
    pulmonary toxicity, 14
    side effects, 14–15
    torsades de pointes, 15
    versus ICDs, 18–19
Amiodarone vs. ICD in Patients with Nonischemic Cardiomyopathy and Asymptomatic Nonsustained VT (AMIOVERT) trial, 52, 71–72
Antiarrhythmic drugs, 18, 19, 49
    interactions with ICDs, 30–31
    sodium channel blocking drugs, 12–13
    used in heart failure, 12–17
    See also Amiodarone; Dofetilide; Sotalol
Antiarrhythmics vs. Implantable Defibrillators (AVID) trial, 18, 20, 35, 36, 64
Arrhythmogenic right ventricular cardiomyopathy, 40–41
Atrial fibrillation, 2, 30, 70–73
    CHF-STAT trial, 70–71
    DIAMOND trial, 72
    management of, 70–73
Atrial flutter, 73–75
    management of, 73–75
    radiofrequency ablation, 74
Antitachycardia pacing, 29
Atrioventricular block, 46, 53–54
Atrioventricular pacing, 25
Atrioventricular synchrony, 64

Biventricular pacing, 65–68
    Multicenter Insync Randomized Clinical Evaluation (MIRACLE) trial, 66–68

Bradyarrhythmias, 13, 61–69
  amiodarone, 15, 61
  causes, 61–62
  conduction system disease, 61
  electromechanical dissociation, 8–9
  implanted defibrillator, 61–63
  pacing for See Bradycardia pacing
Bradycardia pacing
  dual chamber AV versus single chamber ventricular, 63–65
  with ICDs, 25–26, 61–63
  versus ICDs, 61–63
Bundle branch reentry, 39–40
  catheter ablation for, 39–40
  ICDs and, 40

Canadian Implantable Defibrillator Study (CIDS) trial, 20, 23–24, 35
Canadian Trial of Physiologic Pacing (CTOPP), 63–64
Cardiac Arrest Study of Hamburg (CASH) trial, 20, 35
Cardiac arrest survival, 32–36
  ICDs, 32
  patient evaluation, 32–34
  primary cardiac arrest, 35–36
  secondary cardiac arrest, 36
  termination of ventricular tachycardia/fibrillation, 32
  ventricular fibrillation, 33
Cardiac resynchronization therapy (CRT), 67–68
  beta-blockers, 67
  Multicenter Insync Randomized Clinical Evaluation (MIRACLE) trial, 67–68
Cardiomyopathy
  arrhythmogenic right ventricular, 40–41
  ischemic, 1, 2, 4–5, 7, 59
  nonischemic dilated, 1, 5, 7
Catheter ablation, 42, 72, 74
  bundle branch reentry, 39–40
CHF-STAT (Survival Trial of Antiarrhythmic Therapy in Congestive Heart Failure), 47–48, 52, 70–71
Chronic dilated heart failure, 1

Index   105

   Multicenter Insync Randomized Clinical Evaluation (MIRACLE) trial, 66–68
   sudden death in, 9–10
Conduction system disease and bradyarrhythmias, 61
Coronary Artery Bypass Graft (CABG) Patch trial, 49, 50

Danish Investigation of Arrhythmia and Mortality on Dofetilide (DIAMOND) trial, 15–16, 72
Depressed left ventricular function, 45–46
Digoxin, 72
Dofetilide, 3–4, 15–16
   atrial fibrillation and flutter, 15, 72

Electrolyte abnormalities, 8
Electrophysiological study (EPS)
   syncope, 58–59
   with programmed stimulation, 51

Grupo de Estudio de la Sobrevida en la Insuficienca Cardiaca en Argentina (GESICA) trial, 47–48, 51–52

Heart failure
   and atrial fibrillation and flutter, 71–75
   and biventricular pacing, 65–68
   cardiac arrest, 34
   cardiac resynchronization therapy, 67–68
   causes, 1–11
   severity, 19–25, 50
   syndromes, relation of to sudden death, 1–11
   See also Sudden death; Implantable cardioverter-defibrillators (ICDs)

Heart rate variability, 6, 46, 52–53
Hypertrophy and slow ventricular conduction, 3, 4

Idiopathic nonischemic cardiomyopathy
   and lack of scar or infarction, 5
   See also Nonischemic dilated cardiomyopathy
Idiopathic ventricular tachycardia, 40, 41–42, 43

Implantable cardioverter-defibrillators (ICDs), 18–31, 32, 33, 43, 44, 46, 48–52
  advantages over antiarrhythmic drug therapy, 18–19
  antiarrhythmic drug interactions, 30–31
  bradycardia pacing, 25–26, 61–63
  complications, 26–28
  disabling, temporarily, 29–30
  first-line therapy for cardiac arrest survivors, 35–36
  follow-up care, 28–30
  indications, 18–25
  monomorphic ventricular tachycardia, 43
  patient selection, 19–25
  perioperative considerations, 26–28
  psychological support, 31
  risks, minimizing, 26–28
  syncope, 58
  torsades de pointes, 4, 44
  trials, 20, 21–25, 48–51
  unexplained syncope, 18, 59, 60
  versus amiodarone, 18, 48–52
Ischemic cardiomyopathy, 1, 2, 4–5, 7, 19, 59

Monomorphic ventricular tachycardia, 37–42
  arrhythmogenic right ventricular cardiomyopathy, 40–41
  bundle branch reentry, 39–40
  ICD, 40
  long-term therapy for, 42
  scars and, 37
Multicenter Automatic Defibrillator Implantation (MADIT) trial, 49–51
Multicenter Insync Randomized Clinical Evaluation (MIRACLE) trial
  biventricular pacing, 66–68
  cardiac resynchronization therapy (CRT), 67–68
  results, 68
Multicenter Unsustained Tachycardia Trial (MUSTT), 48–49, 51
Myocardial ischemia, 6–7

Nonischemic dilated cardiomyopathy, 1, 5, 7, 39
Nonsustained ventricular tachycardia

CHF-STAT trial, 47–48, 52
heart rate variability, 46, 52–53
in patients with prior myocardial infarction, 48–49
in patients with nonischemic cardiomyopathy, 51–52
marker of sudden death, 46, 47–52
ventricular ectopic activity, 47–48

Pacing
antitachycardia, 29
biventricular, 65–68
bradycardia, 25–26, 61–69
dedicated bradycardia pacing versus ICD, 61–63
dual chamber AV versus single chamber ventricular, 63–65
Polymorphic ventricular tachycardia, 37
and torsades de pointes, 43–44
Potassium and magnesium depletion and torsades de pointes, 3
Prevention of arrhythmic sudden death, 8, 45–55
Primary Progressive Multiple Sclerosis Patients (PROMISE) trial, 47–48
Pulmonary toxicity, amiodarone-induced, 14

Quinidine, 12
QRS
complex, 5
duration, 41, 67–68, 69
morphology in ventricular tachycardia, 39
QT interval, 54–55
and antiarrhythmic drugs, 4, 12, 15–16
beat-to-beat variability, 54–55
prolonged, 4, 12, 15–16, 44, 58
T-wave alternans, 46, 55

Randomized Evaluation of Mechanical Assistance in Congestive Heart Failure (REMATCH) trial, 5
Reentrant ventricular tachycardia
ventricular scars and infarcts as cause of, 4–6
Repolarization and torsades de pointes, 2–4
Risk markers for sudden death
analysis of ST-T and QT interval, 54–55
atrioventricular block, 53–54

Risk markers for sudden death (*Continued*)
    depressed left ventricular function, 45–46
    heart rate variability, 52–53
    nonsustained ventricular tachycardia and ventricular ectopic activity, 47–48
    nonsustained ventricular tachycardia in patients with prior myocardial infarction, 48–51
    nonsustained ventricular tachycardia in patients with non-ischemic cardiomyopathy, 51–52
    secondary cardiac arrest, 36
    syncope, 56
    T-wave alternans, 55

Scars *See* Ventricular scars and infarcts
Slow ventricular conduction and hypertrophy, 4
Sodium channel blocking drugs, 12–13
Sotalol, 16, 71
    atrial fibrillation and flutter, 72
    cause of torsades de pointes, 16
ST-T and QT interval analyses, 54–55
Sudden death
    arrhythmogenic right ventricular cardiomyopathy, 41
    chronic dilated heart failure, 9–10
    heart failure, causes of, 1–11
    implications of multiple causes, 10–11
    myocardial ischemia, 6–7
    prevention of, 8, 10–11, 20, 21, 45–55
    secondary cardiac arrest, 36
    syncope, 56
    therapies to reduce risk of, 8, 10–11, 45–55
    See also Prevention of arrhythmic sudden death; Risk markers for sudden death
Sustained ventricular tachycardia, 37–44
    arrhythmogenic right ventricular cardiomyopathy, 40–41
    bundle branch reentry, 39–40
    idiopathic ventricular tachycardia, 41–42
    monomorphic ventricular tachycardia, 37–43
    polymorphic ventricular tachycardia, 43–44
    therapy for, 42–43
    torsades de pointes, 43–44

Sympathetic stimulation, 6
Syncope, 52
  differential diagnosis, 57
  electrocardiographic abnormalities, 58
  electrophysiological study, 58–59
  ICDs, 58, 59, 60
  initial evaluation and history, 56–58
  long-term ECG monitoring, 58
  unexplained, 18, 59, 60

Thyroid
  and amiodarone, 14
Torsades de pointes, 54
  amiodarone, 15
  causes of, 3–4
  chronic diuretic therapy, 3
  ICD, 43
  polymorphic ventricular tachycardia, 43–44
  potassium and magnesium depletion, 3
  prolonged QT interval, 4, 12, 15–16, 44
  repolarization, 2–4
  sotalol, 15
  susceptibility to, 4, 44, 54
T-wave alternans, 55

Ventricular arrhythmia mechanisms and clinical presentations, 2–9
  repolarization and torsades de pointes, 2–4
Ventricular ectopic activity, 47–48
Ventricular fibrillation, 33
Ventricular hypertrophy, 2–4
  electrophysiologic changes, 3
Ventricular resynchronization
  biventricular pacing, 65–66
  cardiac resynchronization therapy (CRT), 67–68
  Multicenter Insync Randomized Clinical Evaluation (MIRACLE) trial, 66–68
Ventricular scars and infarcts, 1, 41, 51
  bundle branch block reentry, 39
  cause of reentrant ventricular tachycardia, 4–6

Ventricular scars and infarcts (*Continued*)
    cause of monomorphic ventricular tachycardia, 37
    lack of in idiopathic nonischemic cardiomyopathy, 5
Ventricular tachycardia, polymorphic
    See Polymorphic ventricular tachycardia
Ventricular tachycardia, monomorphic
    See Monomorphic ventricular tachycardia
Ventricular tachycardia, sustained
    See Sustained ventricular tachycardia

Sympathetic stimulation, 6
Syncope, 52
 differential diagnosis, 57
 electrocardiographic abnormalities, 58
 electrophysiological study, 58–59
 ICDs, 58, 59, 60
 initial evaluation and history, 56–58
 long-term ECG monitoring, 58
 unexplained, 18, 59, 60

Thyroid
 and amiodarone, 14
Torsades de pointes, 54
 amiodarone, 15
 causes of, 3–4
 chronic diuretic therapy, 3
 ICD, 43
 polymorphic ventricular tachycardia, 43–44
 potassium and magnesium depletion, 3
 prolonged QT interval, 4, 12, 15–16, 44
 repolarization, 2–4
 sotalol, 15
 susceptibility to, 4, 44, 54
T-wave alternans, 55

Ventricular arrhythmia mechanisms and clinical presentations, 2–9
 repolarization and torsades de pointes, 2–4
Ventricular ectopic activity, 47–48
Ventricular fibrillation, 33
Ventricular hypertrophy, 2–4
 electrophysiologic changes, 3
Ventricular resynchronization
 biventricular pacing, 65–66
 cardiac resynchronization therapy (CRT), 67–68
 Multicenter Insync Randomized Clinical Evaluation (MIRACLE) trial, 66–68
Ventricular scars and infarcts, 1, 41, 51
 bundle branch block reentry, 39
 cause of reentrant ventricular tachycardia, 4–6

Ventricular scars and infarcts (*Continued*)
    cause of monomorphic ventricular tachycardia, 37
    lack of in idiopathic nonischemic cardiomyopathy, 5
Ventricular tachycardia, polymorphic
    See Polymorphic ventricular tachycardia
Ventricular tachycardia, monomorphic
    See Monomorphic ventricular tachycardia
Ventricular tachycardia, sustained
    See Sustained ventricular tachycardia